Voice-related Biomarkers

Mette Pedersen • Neveen Hassan Nashaat
Valentina Camesasca
Ramón Hernández Villoria • Sneha Das
Editors

Voice-related Biomarkers

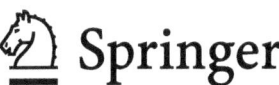

Editors
Mette Pedersen
The Medical Center
Copenhagen, Denmark

Valentina Camesasca
Grande Ospedale Metropolitano Niguarda
Centro Clinico NEMO (NeuroMuscolar
Omnicenter)
Milano, Italy

Sneha Das
Technical University of Denmark
Kongens Lyngby, Denmark

Pioneer Centre for Artificial Intelligence
Copenhagen, Denmark

Neveen Hassan Nashaat
Research on Children with Special Needs
Department
Medical Research and Clinical Studies
Institute
National Research Centre
Cairo, Egypt

Ramón Hernández Villoria
Centro Clínico de Audición y
Lenguaje Cealca
Caracas, Venezuela

Hospital de Clínicas Caracas
Caracas, Venezuela

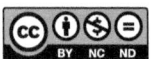

ISBN 978-3-032-03133-4   ISBN 978-3-032-03134-1   (eBook)
https://doi.org/10.1007/978-3-032-03134-1

This work was supported by Mette Pedersen.

© The Editor(s) (if applicable) and The Author(s), under exclusive license to Springer Nature Switzerland AG 2026. This book is an open access publication.

Open Access   This book is licensed under the terms of the Creative Commons Attribution-NonCommercial-NoDerivatives 4.0 International License (http://creativecommons.org/licenses/by-nc-nd/4.0/), which permits any noncommercial use, sharing, distribution and reproduction in any medium or format, as long as you give appropriate credit to the original author(s) and the source, provide a link to the Creative Commons license and indicate if you modified the licensed material. You do not have permission under this license to share adapted material derived from this book or parts of it.

The images or other third party material in this book are included in the book's Creative Commons license, unless indicated otherwise in a credit line to the material. If material is not included in the book's Creative Commons license and your intended use is not permitted by statutory regulation or exceeds the permitted use, you will need to obtain permission directly from the copyright holder.

This work is subject to copyright. All commercial rights are reserved by the author(s), whether the whole or part of the material is concerned, specifically the rights of translation, reprinting, reuse of illustrations, recitation, broadcasting, reproduction on microfilms or in any other physical way, and transmission or information storage and retrieval, electronic adaptation, computer software, or by similar or dissimilar methodology now known or hereafter developed. Regarding these commercial rights a non-exclusive license has been granted to the publisher.

The use of general descriptive names, registered names, trademarks, service marks, etc. in this publication does not imply, even in the absence of a specific statement, that such names are exempt from the relevant protective laws and regulations and therefore free for general use.

The publisher, the authors and the editors are safe to assume that the advice and information in this book are believed to be true and accurate at the date of publication. Neither the publisher nor the authors or the editors give a warranty, expressed or implied, with respect to the material contained herein or for any errors or omissions that may have been made. The publisher remains neutral with regard to jurisdictional claims in published maps and institutional affiliations.

This Springer imprint is published by the registered company Springer Nature Switzerland AG
The registered company address is: Gewerbestrasse 11, 6330 Cham, Switzerland

If disposing of this product, please recycle the paper.

Preface

This book is based on the Zoom meetings of a committee of the Union of European Phoniatricians named Committee on Biomarkers in Phoniatrics, which had its first Zoom meeting on 21 June 2023. Thereafter, there was a Zoom meeting every second month.

At the first Zoom meeting, there was a presentation by Mieke Moerman on the definition of Biomarkers in Phoniatrics. The zoom presentations of this committee highlighted the importance of biomarkers and the use of artificial intelligence in enhancing the early diagnosis and management of pathological voice changes.

The idea has been to reconstruct the Zoom presentations into chapters in this book. Based on the idea of what a book could represent, the Committee on Biomarkers in Phoniatrics accepted in November 2023 a proposal from the subgroup, including well-recognized phoniatricians and engineers, for position statements, and decided to make an application to create a book with Springer publisher. Since it was early in the process, we were mandated to make an estimate of what the topics for the chapters should be. The result is a good collaboration between the editors and the other participants of the Committee for Biomarkers in Phoniatrics.

The chapters include an abstract and an introduction. In the introduction, the literature on the subjects has carefully been followed up to date by the authors. The main part of the chapters includes the perspectives based on the PowerPoint presentations. The discussions elaborated the perspectives. The conclusions are a combination of the author's and the presenter's views.

All figures in this book include AI generated ALT text to support screen-reader accessibility. Christian Frederik Larsen has helped us organize the chapters for the template for the book.

Copenhagen, Denmark	Mette Pedersen
Dokki, Egypt	Neveen Hassan Nashaat
Milano, Italy	Valentina Camesasca
Caracas, Venezuela	Ramón Hernández Villoria
Kongens Lyngby, Denmark	Sneha Das

Contents

Part I Methods

1. **Committee on Biomarkers in Phoniatrics: Introduction** 3
   Mieke Moerman and Valentina Camesasca

2. **Overview of Voice-Related Parameters in Parkinson's Disease: Aspects of Biomarkers** 11
   Mette Pedersen and Vitus Girelli Meiner

3. **AI-Enhanced Voice Analysis for Neurological Diseases** 25
   Neveen Hassan Nashaat

4. **Modeling a Preclinical Screening Tool Based on Voice-Related Biomarkers: The Case of Parkinson's Disease** 39
   Ramón Hernández-Villoria

5. **Glottal Inverse Filtering and Its Application in the Automatic Classification of Diseases from Speech** 53
   Paavo Alku, Ramón Hernández-Villoria, and Sneha Das

6. **AI Models for Voice Disorders: Considerations from Development to Deployment** 73
   Sneha Das

7. **Voice-Related Biomarkers** 87
   Mieke Moerman and Mette Pedersen

8. **Software and Apps for Glottal Inverse Filtering** 95
   Ramón Hernández-Villoria

9. **Quality Evaluation of Voice AI Software** 109
   Sneha Das

Part II Clinical Applications

10 Pathology of Voice-Related Biomarkers in Laryngology 121
Neveen Hassan Nashaat

11 Neurodegenerative Diseases: Aspects of Voice-Related Biomarkers 139
Valentina Camesasca

12 Genetics and the Application of Voice-Related Biomarkers 151
Mette Pedersen and Neveen Hassan Nashaat

13 Optical Coherence Tomography and Voice-Related Biomarkers 161
Mette Pedersen

14 Overview and Conclusion. 175
Mette Pedersen, Neveen Hassan Nashaat,
Ramón Hernández-Villoria, Valentina Camesasca,
and Sneha Das

Contributors

Editors

Mette Pedersen The Medical Center, Copenhagen, Denmark

Valentina Camesasca Grande Ospedale Metropolitano Niguarda, Centro Clinico NEMO (NeuroMuscolar Omnicenter), Milano, Italy

Neveen Hassan Nashaat Research on Children with Special Needs Department, Medical Research and Clinical Studies Institute, National Research Centre, Cairo, Egypt

Ramón Hernández Villoria Centro Clínico de Audición y Lenguaje Cealca, Caracas, Venezuela

Hospital de Clínicas Caracas, Caracas, Venezuela

Sneha Das Technical University of Denmark, Kongens Lyngby, Denmark

Pioneer Centre for Artificial Intelligence, Copenhagen, Denmark

Authors

Paavo Alku Department of Information and Communications Engineering, Aalto University, Espoo, Finland

Valentina Camesasca Grande Ospedale Metropolitano Niguarda, Centro Clinico NEMO (NeuroMuscolar Omnicenter), Milano, Italy

Sneha Das Technical University of Denmark, Kongens Lyngby, Denmark

Pioneer Centre for Artificial Intelligence, Copenhagen, Denmark

Neveen Hassan Nashaat Research on Children with Special Needs Department, Medical Research and Clinical Studies Institute, National Research Centre, Cairo, Egypt

Ramón Hernández-Villoria Centro Clínico de Audición y Lenguaje Cealca, Caracas, Venezuela

Hospital de Clínicas Caracas, Caracas, Venezuela

Vitus Girelli Meiner IT-University, Copenhagen, Denmark

Mieke Moerman Board Member UEP/EAP, TelePHON.digital BV, Founder UEP Biomarkers Committee, St Martens Latem, Belgium

Mette Pedersen The Medical Center, Copenhagen, Denmark

Part I
Methods

Committee on Biomarkers in Phoniatrics: Introduction

Mieke Moerman and Valentina Camesasca

1.1 Introduction

1.1.1 What Are Biomarkers

The term "biomarker" refers to a wide spectrum of medical signs, which can be measured accurately and reproducibly. There are several definitions of biological markers in the literature. In 1998, the National Institutes of Health Biomarkers Definitions Working Group defined a biomarker as "a characteristic that is objectively measured and evaluated as an indicator of normal biological processes, pathogenic processes, or pharmacologic responses to a therapeutic intervention" [1]. The International Program on Chemical Safety, led by the World Health Organization (WHO) and in coordination with the United Nations and the International Labour Organization, defined a biomarker as "any substance, structure, or process that can be measured in the body or its products and influence or predict the incidence of outcome of disease" [2]. In their report on the validity of biomarkers in environmental risk assessment, the WHO stated that the definition of biomarkers needs to include "almost any measurement reflecting an interaction between a biological system and a potential hazard, which may be chemical, physical, or biological. The measured response may be functional and physiological, biochemical at the cellular level, or a molecular interaction" [3].

Biomarkers are by definition objective and quantifiable characteristics (biochemical, radiological, genetic, epigenetic, etc.) of biological processes, but they do not

---

M. Moerman
Board Member UEP/EAP, TelePHON.digital BV, Founder UEP Biomarkers Committee, St Martens Latem, Belgium

V. Camesasca (✉)
Grande Ospedale Metropolitano Niguarda, Centro Clinico NEMO (NeuroMuscolar Omnicenter), Milano, Italy
e-mail: valentina.camesasca@ospedaleniguarda.it

© The Author(s) 2026
M. Pedersen et al. (eds.), *Voice-related Biomarkers*,
https://doi.org/10.1007/978-3-032-03134-1_1

necessarily correlate with a patient's experience of well-being and do not certainly correspond to the patient's clinical state of health or its changes [4]. Although biomarkers' use in clinical research and practice has become so commonplace that they are often considered primary endpoints in trials, there is still confusion about their engagement because of their complexity. For this reason, a joint task force was formed to forge common definitions and to make them publicly available through a continuously updated online document: the "Biomarkers, Endpoints, and other Tools" (BEST) resource [5]. Biomarkers should be distinct from direct measures of how a person feels, functions, or survives.

The worst error we can make is to assume that a correlation between a biomarker and a clinical outcome means that the biomarker constitutes a valid surrogate. We can consider surrogate endpoints only a small subset of well-characterized biomarkers, with well-evaluated clinical relevance, and with statistical inference between their changes and outcomes. To be used in clinical trials, a biomarker needs to reliably, precisely, and repeatably predict a clinical outcome (either benefit or harm) at a low cost, and it requires the determination of relevance, validity, and accuracy [4, 6].

We need to completely understand the normal physiology and pathophysiology of a biological process in a specific disease to consider a biomarker as a surrogate endpoint. Therefore, understanding the relationship between biomarkers and clinical outcomes is necessary to expand their use in clinical practice [4].

1.1.2 What Is Phoniatrics

Phoniatrics, or phoniatry, is the medical discipline related to the normal, pathological, and professional processes of communication (voice, speech, language, and hearing) and swallowing. It is related to all the organs involved in these functions: the mouth, throat (larynx), ears, nose, neck, lungs, and brain. Phoniatrics is a specific discipline, but it also combines the accumulation of knowledge from both medical and nonmedical fields of science.

The field of voice studies acoustic and aerodynamic parameters and the biomechanics of articulation and resonance. It ranges from voice training to vocal ergonomics and from vocal hygiene to the complex neurologic, psychiatric, and sociological basis of interpersonal communication.

Concerning speech and language disorders, phoniatrics evaluates the motor function of vocal cords, tongue, mouth, and pharynx, as well as nasalance and intelligibility, psychomotor, cognitive, and auditory function, and it provides preventive counseling, speech therapy, and medical or surgical treatment.

Phoniatrics also evaluates the swallowing function. Through endoscopic and/or radiological examination, it analyzes possible drooling, retention, regurgitation, penetration, and aspiration, and it finds adequate rehabilitation and interventions to prevent dehydration, malnutrition, respiratory events, and even death.

Finally, phoniatrics studies the physiology and pathology of hearing through several tests, and it offers different aids, including medical and surgical treatments [7].

1.1.3 Glottal Function: Voice and Swallowing

The larynx has a special position in the middle of the neck, at the crossroads of the upper aerodigestive tracts. Therefore, the glottis has three important and highly relevant functions: breathing, phonation, and airway protection during swallowing. In fact, it is regulated by a complex mechanism that makes it open during ventilation, closed during swallowing, and modulates airflow passage during phonation with vocal fold vibration.

The prevalence of dysphagia and dysphonia is 4% and 3%–9%, respectively, in the adult population. Voice and swallowing disorders are much more frequent in special conditions: they are found in 80% of patients with Parkinson's disease, in 84%–93% of patients with Alzheimer's disease, and in about 40% of patients with head and neck cancer.

Therefore, it is necessary to investigate the pathophysiology underlying dysphagia and dysphonia in specific diseases for obtaining possible biomarkers to diagnose, monitor, and predict outcomes in different disorders.

1.2 Perspectives

1.2.1 Biomarkers in Phoniatrics

As previously stated, in recent years, there has been a growing interest in biomarkers in clinical research and in clinical practice. Recent advances in data science have set the stage for the emergence of new "omics," that is, data science subfields founded on a large amount of data representing the structure or function of a biological system [8]. Biomarkers related to voice, speech, swallowing, and hearing could provide important clinical insights into patients' health status, but they need to ensure sensitivity. If so, they could be useful in screening, diagnosis, remote monitoring, and the development of new surrogate endpoints for clinical trials. We still have almost no biomarkers related to swallowing, just some biomarkers related to hearing, but a more significant number of biomarkers related to voice because of their noninvasive, accessible, and low-cost collection and recording capability via computers or smartphones [8].

1.2.2 Voice-Related Biomarkers

The voice-related biomarker is a signature, a feature, or a combination of features from, among others, the audio signal of the voice that is associated with a clinical outcome and can be used to monitor patients, diagnose a condition, or grade the severity or the stages of a disease [9, 10]. The development of new technology, such as artificial intelligence (AI) and machine learning (a branch of AI able to learn and adapt without following explicit instructions by using predictive algorithms and statistical models to analyze and draw inferences from patterns in data), allows for efficient analysis of voice data and makes it possible to discover voice-related biomarkers. In this technological era, patients' audio recordings are being investigated as possible digital biomarkers for the early detection of a broad range of conditions [8]. Some of the cohorts of highest interest include neurological disorders (such as Parkinson's disease and Alzheimer's disease), mood disorders (such as generalized anxiety disorder and major depressive disorder), cardiorespiratory disorders (such as COVID-19 and congestive heart failure), pediatric disorders (such as Friedreich's ataxia and autism spectrum disorder), and other voice disorders (such as laryngeal cancers and benign lesions) [10].

Changes in voice features are found in up to 78% of patients with early-stage Parkinson's disease, and they are mostly related to phonation and articulation, including pitch variations, decreased energy in the higher parts of the harmonic spectrum, and imprecise articulation of vowels and consonants, leading to decreased intelligibility [9]. Subtle voice modifications can be detected even years before the typical prodromal symptoms of Alzheimer's disease and cognitive impairment; they mainly concern verbal fluency [9]. Voice impairment and dysarthria are frequently perceived in multiple sclerosis and neuromuscular disorders, and they can correlate with the progression of disease. Patients with chronic inflammatory disorders (such as rheumatoid arthritis and systemic lupus erythematosus), chronic autoimmune connective tissue disorders (such as systemic sclerosis and Sjogren syndrome), and endocrine disorders (such as diabetes mellitus and hypothyroidism) may present voice feature modifications due to the pathological changes in the larynx, which significantly correlate with biochemical parameters of inflammation and hormonal status [9, 11]. Patients with cardiovascular disease may also have voice alterations through the systemic process of atherosclerosis; in fact, it may lead to chronic hypoperfusion of the larynx and other organs and neurologic structures involved in phonation, determining structural changes with consequent incomplete closure of the vocal folds, reduced laryngeal mobility, reduced cartilage sliding, decreased mucosal wave vibration, and therefore predictable changes in voice features [11]. Finally, modifications of voice characteristics may correlate with respiratory diseases (especially COVID-19 and acute respiratory illness), mental health (psychiatric and behavioral disorders), and mood disorders (anxiety and depression) [9, 11].

In light of the above conditions, we can state that the human voice offers the unique opportunity to capture subtle physiological and pathological changes associated with human health [10]. However, voice feature changes do not probably reflect glottal function; acoustics alone are not sufficient. Human voice production depends on the synchronized cooperation of multiple physiological systems, which makes the voice sensitive to changes [12]. This process requires the complex cooperation of the lungs, which provide the air pressure; the larynx, in which vocal fold vibrations modulate airflow passage, producing a sound; and the vocal tract (the area from the top of the larynx to the lips that contains articulators including the tongue, jaw, and soft palate), which further filters sound spreading (resonance) and determines the final vocal product. Moreover, voice is different from speech and language. Speech refers to a primary mode of expressing thoughts, ideas, emotions, or information between individuals by the articulation of sounds through the vocal tract [10]. Language is created by cognition and linguistic knowledge. It involves the production of speech sounds into meaningful units (phonology), the combination of these meaningful units into words, and the generation of sentences and paragraphs to communicate thought [11]. Nevertheless, voice can provide a sensitive snapshot of cognition, tissue integrity, and motor function relevant to many diseases, because it reflects the coordination of a variety of cognitive and motor processes [11].

A good voice-related biomarker should be specific for disease groups, independent of age, and independent of language, accent, or culture-specific features and geographic location. It should be noninvasive, nonintrusive, acquired remotely, and in a short period of time. Voice-related biomarkers should be combined with other digital technologies and integrated into the electronic medical record with established clinical protocols and practice patterns in a secure and encrypted way [9, 11].

Presumably, AI is needed to determine the weight of the different dimensions and to obtain accurate digital voice-related biomarkers. The first step would be to develop standards for their collection and create large-scale voice sample data stores for clinical use. This should be followed by integrating the algorithm into a user-friendly device (smartphone app, smart home device, etc.), because it won't be the algorithm alone but its embedding in a connected medical device, which will be approved by the agencies [9]. No current AI technology investigating voice as a biomarker of health is currently approved by the FDA [10]. We need to get a proper evaluation of usability, adaptability, efficacy, and safety, but we also have to consider the sociological and ethical implications of using voice-related biomarkers and voice technologies [9]. Therefore, it is strongly recommended to establish a large dataset of labeled audios associated with clinical outcomes, to combine that into algorithms of digital devices, and to run prospective randomized controlled trials and real-world evaluations before envisaging voice-related biomarker scale-up [9].

1.2.3 Biomarker Committee of the Union of European Phoniatricians (UEP)

In the evolving landscape of voice-related biomarkers of human health, laryngologists will be at the forefront. These professionals are the experts in laryngeal anatomy and function and the ones who better understand the physiological processes underlying voice changes in different diseases, which means they possess the knowledge to be critical in the development of technology connected to voice-related biomarkers [10].

The UEP Biomarker Committee started its activities in 2023 under the leadership of Professor Mieke Moerman. It encompasses a group of medical doctors, ENT specialists, and phoniatricians from different parts of the world and with different dispositions. The aim of the Committee is to develop knowledge about biomarkers regarding voice in different disorders.

It was decided that the first target population would be Parkinson's disease and that the voice function would be first analyzed. However, as previously stated, voice changes do not necessarily reflect glottal function; the voice is multi-dimensional. The three most important and relevant functions of the glottis are breathing, phonation, and protection of the airways during swallowing, and they focus primarily on the vocal fold closure. Indeed, worthy glottal closure is not only necessary for a good voice but also to prevent aspiration and pulmonary complications. For that reason, the committee decided to work on defining (and ultimately testing) biomarkers that reveal the glottal function and to explore the possibility of obtaining reliable tests related to glottal closure, including aerodynamic voice dimension, also via inverse filtering of the voice signal.

1.3 Discussion

The voice is a gorgeous medium that serves as a primary source of communication between individuals. It is one of the most natural, energy-efficient ways of interacting with each other [9]. The dynamic, typical qualities of the human voice are strongly influenced by different physiological states and can detect subtle pathological changes associated with human health. Therefore, the human voice offers the unique opportunity for developing specialized digital biomarkers and enabling objective and noninvasive screening, diagnosis, and monitoring of several health conditions [10].

The evolution of voice-related tests and technology, audio signal analysis, and natural language processing methods has opened the way to numerous potential applications of voice, such as the identification of voice-related biomarkers for diagnosis, classification, or patient remote monitoring [9]. Voice-related biomarkers are tremendously spreading because of their noninvasive, accessible, and low-cost collection and recording capability via computers or smartphones [8]. The US Food and Drug Administration (FDA) and the National Institute of Health created a Biomarkers, Endpoints, and other Tools (BEST) glossary, within which they defined a biomarker as "a characteristic that is measured as an indicator of normal biological processes, pathogenic processes, or biological responses to an exposure or intervention, including therapeutic interventions" [5]. Before 2013, there were a total of 81 publications in PubMed relating to voice as a biomarker of health. Between 2014 and 2018, there were 122 publications, and the last 5 years saw 240 publications on the topic. According to a study performed by Brand Essence Research in 2022, the financial investment made in the field of voice-related biomarkers was worth USD 1.9B in 2021 and is projected to exceed USD 5.1B by 2028, for a compound annual growth rate of 15.15% [10]. In recent years, the BEST definition has encompassed digital biomarkers, which refer to measures or features collected by digital health technologies, sharing the same characteristics and objectives as traditional biomarkers mentioned above [8, 10, 12]. The advancement of digital biomarkers and the development of remote health care have greatly progressed during the global COVID-19 pandemic. Combining voice and speech data with artificial intelligence and machine-based learning offers a novel solution to the growing demand for telemedicine [11]. Being so sensitive, voice features could open possibilities for earlier diagnosis of several disorders affecting voice through the use of voice-related biomarkers [12]. Since the collection of acoustic data is a noninvasive process that can be performed at a low cost, the voice as a digital biomarker could be a diagnostic and prognostic resource with the potential to be a more economical and ecological measure for the assessment of health [12].

Although the future of voice-related biomarkers is promising, there remain important limitations to broad integration into clinical care because of the lack of standards in how to collect voice data and the lack of prospective studies and validation of AI algorithms [8]. Determining voice-related biomarkers should be simple and straightforward, affordable, largely accessible, and available. It needs quality control by continuous resampling to ensure high-quality verified recordings and reduce detection errors [11]. The development of voice-related biomarkers, with proven validity and reliability, needs greater standardization in voice data collection and analysis protocols to gain large datasets labeled with clinical outcomes. It is necessary to make a systematic and rigorous evaluation of voice-related biomarkers in demographically and linguistically diverse populations from different geographic regions and large prospective clinical trials evaluating the use of voice as surrogate endpoints of disease. Because of the lack of established guidelines outlining best practices for remote care, it is advisable to be cautious about false positives and false negatives so as not to rely only on digital biomarkers.

The use of artificial intelligence-derived output in clinical practice implies an understanding of the mechanism linking voice feature changes to disease states since the market is moving from the research and development stage towards commercialization and roll-out of technologies to patients and health care systems [10, 11]. No current AI technology investigating voice as a biomarker of health is currently approved by the FDA [10]. The Biomarker Committee of the Union of European Phoniatricians is a new entity with the aim of developing knowledge about digital technologies regarding characteristics and features in different disorders and defining easily accessible parameters with the potential of leading to a biomarker for glottal closure. The identified voice-related biomarkers should be objectively measurable and serve as indicators of normal biological activities, disease-related processes, or responses to therapeutic treatments.

1.4 Conclusion

There is growing enthusiasm surrounding voice tests and features as possible biomarkers in health care technologies because of their noninvasive, accessible, and low-cost collection capability via computers or smartphones. A more complete understanding of the physiological process in a specific disease and a comprehensive knowledge of the relationship between voice features and clinical outcomes are necessary to consider digital biomarkers as a surrogate and even a true endpoint and to expand their use in clinical practice. More research is needed to accurately achieve the entirety of this field and promote voice-related biomarkers in remote health care.

References

1. Biomarkers Definition Working Group. Biomarkers and surrogate endpoints: preferred definitions and conceptual framework. Clin Pharmacol Ther. 2001;69:89–95. https://doi.org/10.1067/mcp.2001.113989.
2. World Health Organization, International Programme on Chemical Safety. Biomarkers in risk assessment: validity and validation. Geneva: World Health Organization; 2001. Available from: http://www.inchem.org/documents/ehc/ehc/ehc222.htm
3. World Health Organization, International Programme on Chemical Safety. Biomarkers and risk assessment: concepts and principles. Geneva: World Health Organization; 1993. Available from: https://iris.who.int/handle/10665/39037
4. Strimbu K, Tavel JA. What are biomarkers? Curr Opin HIV AIDS. 2010;5:463–6. https://doi.org/10.1097/COH.0b013e32833ed177.
5. FDA-NIH Biomarker Working Group. BEST (Biomarkers, EndpointS, and other tools) resource. Silver Spring/Bethesda: Food and Drug Administration (US)/National Institutes of Health (US); 2016. Available from: https://www.ncbi.nlm.nih.gov/books/NBK326791/
6. Califf RM. Biomarker definitions and their applications. Exp Biol Med (Maywood). 2018;243:213–21. https://doi.org/10.1177/1535370217750088.
7. Oguz H, Hess M, Klein AM. Phoniatrics. Biomed Res Int. 2015;2015:156014. https://doi.org/10.1155/2015/156014.
8. Bensoussan Y, Elemento O, Rameau A. Voice as an AI biomarker of health – introducing audiomics. JAMA Otolaryngol Head Neck Surg. 2024;150:283–4. https://doi.org/10.1001/jamaoto.2023.4807.
9. Fagherazzi G, Fischer A, Ismael M, Despotovic V. Voice for health: the use of vocal biomarkers from research to clinical practice. Digit Biomark. 2021;5:78–88. https://doi.org/10.1159/000515346.
10. Evangelista EG, Bélisle-Pipon JC, Naunheim MR, Powell M, Gallois H, Bensoussan Y, Bridge2AI-Voice Consortium. Voice as a biomarker in health-tech: mapping the evolving landscape of voice biomarkers in the start-up world. Otolaryngol Head Neck Surg. 2024;171:340–52. https://doi.org/10.1002/ohn.830.
11. Sara JDS, Orbelo D, Maor E, Lerman LO, Lerman A. Guess what we can hear – novel voice biomarkers for the remote detection of disease. Mayo Clin Proc. 2023;98:1353–75. https://doi.org/10.1016/j.mayocp.2023.03.007.
12. Idrisoglu A, Dallora AL, Anderberg P, Berglund JS. Applied machine learning techniques to diagnose voice-affecting conditions and disorders: systematic literature review. J Med Internet Res. 2023;25:e46105. https://doi.org/10.2196/46105.

Open Access This chapter is licensed under the terms of the Creative Commons Attribution-NonCommercial-NoDerivatives 4.0 International License (http://creativecommons.org/licenses/by-nc-nd/4.0/), which permits any noncommercial use, sharing, distribution and reproduction in any medium or format, as long as you give appropriate credit to the original author(s) and the source, provide a link to the Creative Commons license and indicate if you modified the licensed material. You do not have permission under this license to share adapted material derived from this chapter or parts of it.

The images or other third party material in this chapter are included in the chapter's Creative Commons license, unless indicated otherwise in a credit line to the material. If material is not included in the chapter's Creative Commons license and your intended use is not permitted by statutory regulation or exceeds the permitted use, you will need to obtain permission directly from the copyright holder.

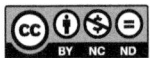

Overview of Voice-Related Parameters in Parkinson's Disease: Aspects of Biomarkers

Mette Pedersen and Vitus Girelli Meiner

2.1 Introduction

Biomarkers are of interest for research and for identifying the most valuable voice-related parameters in the clinic [1]. The identified biomarkers should be objectively measurable and indicate normal biological activities, disease-related processes, or responses to treatments [2]. The National Institute of Health (US) in 1998 defined a biomarker as a characteristic that is objectively measured and evaluated as an indicator of normal biological processes, pathogenic processes, or pharmacological responses to therapeutic interventions. Till now, the discussion is open about which biomarkers can be used in a clinical situation. A discussion based on Mieke Moormann's research concluded with the following test ratings of listeners and subjective complaints: the GRBAS test, the VHI test, and the ratings of acoustic analysis and MPT, referring to a consensus by the Union of European Phoniatricians and the European Laryngological Society. The consensus did not include artificial intelligence evaluation (AI) [3]. (A list of definitions is provided below). Since Parkinson's disease is a big and well-defined area in a library search, the focus was started here for eventual clinical voice-related biomarkers, also including machine learning.

Genetics is a considerable research area for voice-related biomarkers with clinical aspects in the future. A sincere problem is that we have to consider which voice-related biomarkers are usable for genetic research to compare the voice with genes. A paper has till now used around 80 voice parameters taken from an open-access voice analysis system, PRAAT, with a comparison to the genomes of 12,901 Icelanders, where they found a gene related to the fundamental frequency. The weak

M. Pedersen (✉)
The Medical Center, Copenhagen, Denmark
e-mail: M.f.pedersen@dadlnet.dk

V. G. Meiner
IT-University, Copenhagen, Denmark

definition of the voice-related parameters is a problem [4]. In this connection, it is our responsibility as medical doctors and clinicians to help researchers but also firms, for example, the firm O LINK®, that base their development on genetic hardware and software, to give clinical feedback.

It is necessary to acknowledge that without randomized controlled trials documenting the evidence of voice-related biomarkers, they will not be clinically established. This is a difficult area for both measures, with and without AI. There are suggestions for solutions involving AI in the way that the prospective data arm and placebo arm are supplemented with a third technical arm [5]. In this way, AI can be included in randomized controlled trials in a clinically feasible way. Another approach is the Cochrane Library software, capable of sorting out whether papers on voice-related biomarkers are randomized [6, 7].

Concerning voice analysis, biomarkers are very important for many voice-related disorders, not only located in the larynx but also neurological disorders. We looked for papers on voice-related biomarkers for the years 2013–2023. The result showed that the disorder Parkinson's disease included voice analysis to a much greater extent than other disorders. Therefore, we searched for voice-related biomarkers in Parkinson's disease, and here we found, surprisingly, that there is a wealth of articles on AI starting in 2013/2014. It was possible to analyze the literature for voice analyses used in the papers with and without AI (non-AI).

Within the existing literature, there is a notable transition from non-machine learning (non-ML) to machine learning (ML) analyses, complicating the discussion of voice-related biomarkers. The majority of studies on ML are either retrospective or case–control. No prospective randomized controlled trials investigating voice-related biomarkers with AI were identified.

This study aimed, therefore, to evaluate the papers on Parkinson's disease related to voice measures to get an impression of which voice analyses are used in the clinic. From there, a discussion of valid voice-related biomarkers can start, also with the aspect of AI. There is in the literature a mix of voice and speech analysis. Since we are focusing on voice-related biomarkers, speech-related papers have been excluded. We have also excluded the papers where voice function was extracted from running speech, since the relation between voice analysis and speech is inadequately documented.

2.2 Method

The results are based on two literature searches performed by The Royal Society of Medicine Library (UK). In the first one, the search title "Vocal Biomarkers and Artificial Intelligence" was until March 2023. Here, we discovered 332 papers, surprisingly including a significant number focused on Parkinson's disease, with 54 papers specifically addressing this condition.

That is why we focused on "Voice Parameters in Parkinson's Disease" in the second search in August 2023. Since the papers included AI after 2013, we focused on time intervals from 2013 to 2023. The librarians found 98 papers [8–103]. Some of them were reviews.

We constructed a table, concentrating on the era preceding the heavy use of AI and the era of AI. This later phase was primarily characterized by articles focused on AI concepts. Additionally, we have elucidated the insights from the reviews conducted during the analysis period, before and after the emergence of AI.

There was some discussion with the librarians about whether they found all the papers, since with Google, a supplementary eight references were provided. Upon our request, they have reviewed the eight and compared them with the search strategy employed back in August 2023. Of the eight, three were not indexed in Medline or Embase, making them inaccessible through the search strategy utilized. Five references were indeed identified by the search strategy. However, per the instruction to *exclude* 'speech' from the search criteria, these references were not selected for inclusion during the manual review process. The selection criteria focused on "voice parameters (excluding speech) in Parkinson's disease," emphasizing factors such as the harmonics-to-noise ratio (HNR), jitter, shimmer, intensity in decibel (dB) levels, fundamental frequency (F0), and mean phonation time (MPT), as specified. It is underlined that voice function is not the same as speech, and the evaluation methods are different.

2.3 Material

The two searches gave 332 results in the first search. A total of 98 papers were related to Parkinson's disease in the second search. Hereof, the 47 papers were based on 7561 patients (23 papers without patient numbers) and 1513 controls from 2013 to 2019 (minus 5 reviews on non-AI). Between 2013 and 2019, 47 papers had voice-related parameters in Parkinson's disease, of which 4 included Artificial Intelligence (AI). Between 2019 and 2023, 51 papers were related to voice parameters in Parkinson's disease, of which 20 included AI.

Based on the papers, we tried to divide the relevant information on voice-related parameters. The parameters used without machine learning (ML) were markedly different from those in machine learning (ML) papers. When initiating a review, it can be challenging to categorize the importance of various aspects; hence, the summary isn't systematically divided into *tests* and *measurements*. We tried to use the definitions from the literature below.

List with Definitions of Tests and Measurements in the Article
- *Artificial Intelligence*: The simulation of human intelligence processes by machines, especially computer systems.
- *Case/Control Study*: A type of observational study that compares subjects with a specific condition (cases) to those without (controls).
- *Cepstrum Analysis*: A tool used in speech signal processing to measure the periodicity or pitch of a signal.

- *Deep Brain Operation Made*: Refers to surgical interventions in the brain, such as those for treating Parkinson's disease, which may impact vocal function.
- *Deep Learning*: A subset of machine learning based on artificial neural networks that resemble learning.
- *F0 (Fundamental Frequency)*: The lowest frequency of a periodic waveform, representing the pitch of the voice; standard deviation likely refers to a measure of variability or dispersion around the mean (average) value.
- *GRBAS (Grade, Roughness, Breathiness, Asthenia, Strain)*: A scale used by clinicians to subjectively assess voice quality.
- *HNR (Harmonics-to-Noise Ratio)*: A measure used in voice analysis to quantify the amount of harmonic sound to background noise in a voice signal.
- *Intensity Measurements in dB*: The assessment of the loudness of a sound, often used in speech and voice analysis.
- *Inverse filtering:* The process of receiving the input of a system from its output. It is the simplest approach to restore the original image once the degradation function is known.
- *Jitter (ABS/%)*: A measure of frequency variation in the voice (absolute and percent), reflecting stability in pitch production.
- *Laryngoscopy*: A procedure that allows a doctor to look at the back of the throat, larynx, and vocal cords, usually with a scope.
- *Machine Learning*: A subset of artificial intelligence that involves the development of algorithms allowing computers to learn from and make predictions or decisions based on data.
- *MPT (Mean Phonation Time)*: The average duration a person can sustain a vowel sound on one breath, used to assess vocal function.
- *Praat Analysis*: The use of Praat software, a popular tool for analyzing, synthesizing, and manipulating voice, speech, and singing.
- *Prospective Article*: An article that describes a study that follows participants over a planned period of time to observe outcomes.
- *Randomized Parameters*: Variables in a study that are randomly assigned to participants to reduce bias.
- *Retrospective Study*: A study that looks back at data collected in the past to analyze outcomes.
- *Shimmer (ABS/%)*: A measure of amplitude variation in the voice, indicating stability in loudness.
- *SNR (Signal-to-Noise Ratio)*: The ratio of the power of a signal (meaningful information) to the power of background noise.
- *Software*: Programs and other operating information used by a computer.
- *Spectrograms (LTAS—Long-Term Average Spectrum)*: Visual representations of the spectrum of frequencies in a sound or signal as they vary with time.
- *Telephone Analysis*: A method of analyzing voice quality using telephone transmission characteristics; not a standard phoniatric term, may refer to telephony-based voice analysis methods.

- **VHI *(Voice Handicap Index)*:** A questionnaire with scores used to assess a patient's perception of the impact of voice problems on their daily life.
- **VRP *(Voice Range Profile)*:** A graphical representation of the range of pitches and volumes a voice can produce.

2.4 Results

The validation in Table 2.1 is based on 7561 patients (23 papers without patient numbers) and 1513 controls (58 without numbers) (minus reviews). Most studies are on early and moderate cases of Parkinson's disease. A total of 7 papers present the results of deep brain treatment.

Table 2.1 Parameters found in the articles

Parameters	Total
No patient (cases)	7561 (23 without no.)
Prospective articles	25
Randomized articles	5
Retrospective articles	6
Controls	1513
HNR	23
SNR	8
F0 (+ SD)	40
Intensity	24
JITTER ABS/%	29
SHIMMER ABS/%	23
Spektral and LTAS	9
CEPSTRUM analysis	5
VRP	4
VHI	25
MPT	14
GRBAS	10
Deep brain surgery	7
Telephone calls	3
Praat reference	13
AI	24
Deep learning	9
Laryngoscopy	6

The table shows the non-AI voice analysis in the papers; it is noted that fundamental frequency is mostly used. It is noted that in the overview of articles, 24 include AI; they are later discussed. Copyright: Pedersen M (2025) [104], redistributed under the terms of the Creative Commons Attribution License (CC BY 4.0)

Between 2013 and 2019, 47 papers included voice-related parameters in Parkinson's disease; four of these included ML. Between 2019 and 2023, 51 papers had voice parameters in Parkinson's disease, of which 20 included ML. The most used voice parameters in non-ML papers related to Parkinson's disease, with the number of papers in parentheses, were fundamental frequency + standard deviation (40); jitter, absolute, and percent (29); shimmer, absolute, and percent (23); harmonics-to-noise ratio (23); voice handicap index (25); and intensity measurement (24). Other parameters are mentioned up to 14 times: Signal-to-Noise Ratio, Maximum Phonation Time, Spectrography and LTAS, Cepstrum Analysis, Voice Range Profile, and the GRBAS test. Five reviews conducted between 2018 and 2021 on voice-related parameters in Parkinson's disease showed great heterogeneity between studies [44, 49, 62, 64, 95].

Between 2019 and 2023, 51 papers were related to voice parameters in Parkinson's disease, of which 20 included ML. Out of 98, 24 papers included AI, with 6488 cases and 531 controls, using 2–453 features to identify voice-related parameters. Two reviews on data sets, recording protocols, and signal analysis from 2022 and 2023 showed issues with limited, unbalanced, and large differences between data sets [105, 106]. Support Vector Machines were used in nine cases, and deep learning in nine cases. Praat software was used in six cases. It is noticed that the features varied from 2 to 453, which is difficult to handle for the evaluation of eventual voice-related biomarkers (Table 2.2).

In Table 2.2, it was noted that there was a great variability of features. Praat software has two systems, one with and one without machine learning (ML).

Table 2.2 The papers used for this table contain AI/ML (24 papers)

Parameters	Total
No patient (cases)	6488
Controls	531 (6 papers well defined)
Support Vector Machine (SVM)	9—(13 other ML-based)
Features	2–453
Praat software	6
Telephone calls	3

2.5 Discussion and Conclusion

Well-defined features and data sets for ML are essential in the future to measure quantitative deviations of voice, as given with the example of Parkinson's disease, usable as biomarkers, also in AI. The number of patients in the papers in this overview was difficult to estimate, although the measures used were clear from paper to paper. Some papers differentiate between the early and advanced stages of the disease, and some do not. Quantitative validation of the single voice parameters can be done by, e.g., comparing early, moderate, and heavy Parkinson's disease to healthy controls or patients at various ages, at best, also to other disorders. Non-AI papers show clear differences in the measured parameters compared to healthy controls and also to treatment effect, but a comparison between the papers is difficult. Mostly, the studies are not comparable at all, and the results were not quantitatively compared to other disorders, like, e.g., Alzheimer's disease. The artificial intelligence studies had a large variety, especially of features (parameters). A dialog with the ML researchers based on the consensus paper is necessary [3].

References

1. Strimbu K, Tavel JA. What are biomarkers? Curr Opin HIV AIDS. 2010;5:463–6. https://doi.org/10.1097/COH.0b013e32833ed177.
2. Fagherazzi G, Fischer A, Ismael M, Despotovic V. Voice for health: the use of vocal biomarkers from research to clinical practice. Digit Biomark. 2021;5:78–88. https://doi.org/10.1159/000515346.
3. Lechien JR, Geneid A, Bohlender JE, Cantarella G, Avellaneda JC, Desuter G, et al. Consensus for voice quality assessment in clinical practice: guidelines of the European Laryngological Society and Union of the European Phoniatricians. Eur Arch Otorrinolaringol. 2023;280:5459–73. https://doi.org/10.1007/s00405-023-08211-6.
4. Gisladottir RS, Helgason A, Halldorsson BV, Helgason H, Borsky M, Chien YR, et al. Sequence variants affecting voice pitch in humans. Sci Adv. 2023;9:eabq2969. https://doi.org/10.1126/sciadv.abq2969.
5. Lee CS, Lee AY. How artificial intelligence can transform randomized controlled trials. Transl Vis Sci Technol. 2020;9:9. https://doi.org/10.1167/tvst.9.2.9.
6. Marshall IJ, Noel-Storr A, Kuiper J, Thomas J, Wallace BC. Machine learning for identifying randomized controlled trials: an evaluation and practitioner's guide. Res Synth Methods. 2018;9:602–14. https://doi.org/10.1002/jrsm.1287.
7. Higgins JPT, Savović J, Page MJ, Elbers RG, Sterne JAC. Chapter 8: Assessing risk of bias in a randomized trial. In: Higgins JPT, Thomas J, Chandler J, Cumpston M, Li T, Page MJ, et al., Cochrane handbook for systematic reviews of interventions version 6.4 (updated August 2023). Cochrane; 2023. Available from: www.training.cochrane.org/handbook.
8. Louis ED, Gerbin M. Voice handicap in essential tremor: a comparison with normal controls and Parkinson's disease. Tremor Other Hyperkinet Mov (N Y). 2013;3:tre-03-114-970-1. https://doi.org/10.7916/D8KD1WN3.
9. Bauer V, Aleric Z, Janic E, Knežević B, Prpić D, Kaćavenda A. Voice assessment in Parkinson disease and multiple sclerosis patients. Eur Arch Otorrinolaringol. 2012;270:1.
10. Péron J, Cekic S, Haegelen C, Sauleau P, Drapier D, Vérin M, et al. Influence of the relevant acoustic features on the recognition of emotional prosody following subthalamic nucleus deep brain stimulation in Parkinson's disease. Behav Neurol. 2013;27(3):416.

11. Bang YI, Min K, Sohn YH, Cho SR. Acoustic characteristics of vowel sounds in patients with Parkinson disease. NeuroRehabilitation. 2013;32(3):649–54. https://doi.org/10.3233/NRE-130887.
12. Teixeira EG, Howard D, Moffatt S, Miller N, Silbergleit AK, et al. An acoustic and perceptual investigation of speech and voice in Parkinson's and in depression. J Parkinsons Dis. 2013;3(Suppl 1):144.
13. Silbergleit AK, LeWitt PA, Peterson EL, Gardner GM. Quantitative analysis of voice in Parkinson disease compared to motor performance: a pilot study. J Parkinsons Dis. 2015;5(3):517–24. https://doi.org/10.3233/JPD-140526.
14. Jafari A. Classification of Parkinson's disease patients using nonlinear phonetic features and mel-frequency cepstral analysis. Biomed Eng Appl Basis Commun. 2013;25(4) https://doi.org/10.4015/S1016237213500014.
15. Smith LK, Goberman AM. Long-time average spectrum in individuals with Parkinson disease. NeuroRehabilitation. 2014;35(1):77–88. https://doi.org/10.3233/NRE-141102.
16. Yang S, Zheng F, Luo X, Cai S, Wu Y, Liu K, et al. Effective dysphonia detection using feature dimension reduction and kernel density estimation for patients with Parkinson's disease. PLoS One. 2014;9(2):e88825. https://doi.org/10.1371/journal.pone.0088825.
17. Soares DP, Santos FM, Andrade L. Vocal characteristics in subjects with Parkinson's disease. Int Arch Otorhinolaryngol. 2015;19(Suppl 2):S117.
18. Spazzapan EA, Alves E, Fabbron E, Gradim EM, Onofri A, Motonaga SM. Vocal complaints and voice characteristics in individuals with Parkinson disease: a preliminary study. Int Arch Otorhinolaryngol. 2015;19(Suppl 2):S117–8.
19. Tanaka Y, Tsuboi T, Watanabe H, Kajita Y, Fujimoto Y, Ohdake R, et al. Voice features of Parkinson's disease patients with subthalamic nucleus deep brain stimulation. J Neurol. 2015;262(5):1173–81. https://doi.org/10.1007/s00415-015-7681-z.
20. Manor Y, Naor S, Shpunt D, Diamant N, Hillel A, Ezra A, et al. Machine learning classifiers and subjective vocal perception of Parkinson's disease patients and healthy control. Mov Disord. 2019;34(Suppl 2):S394. Available from: https://www.mdsabstracts.org/abstract/machine-learning-classifiers-and-subjective-vocal-perception-of-parkinsons-disease-patients-and-healthy-control/
21. Tsuboi T, Watanabe H, Tanaka Y, Ohdake R, Yoneyama N, Hara K, et al. Characteristic laryngoscopic findings in Parkinson's disease patients after subthalamic nucleus deep brain stimulation and its correlation with voice disorder. J Neural Transm (Vienna). 2015;122(12):1663–72. https://doi.org/10.1007/s00702-015-1436-y.
22. Crino C, Palmer A, Bryans LA, Graville DJ. Characteristics associated with voice handicap in Parkinson's disease. J Parkinsons Dis. 2016;6(Suppl 1):110.
23. Watts CR. A retrospective study of long-term treatment outcomes for reduced vocal intensity in hypokinetic dysarthria. BMC Ear Nose Throat Disord. 2016;16:2. https://doi.org/10.1186/s12901-016-0022-8.
24. Postuma RB. Voice changes in prodromal Parkinson's disease: is a new biomarker within earshot? Sleep Med. 2016;19:148–9. https://doi.org/10.1016/j.sleep.2015.08.019.
25. Gillivan-Murphy P, Colreavy M. Vocal tract tremor in Parkinson's disease. Ir J Med Sci. 2016;185(Suppl 3):S160.
26. Abrahao L, Marques C, Lemme E. Swallowing and voice assessment by manofluorography in patients with Parkinson's disease. Gastroenterology. 2016;150(6 Suppl 1):S862–3. https://doi.org/10.1016/S0016-5085(16)32906-7.
27. Cannito MP, Ramig LO, Halpern AE, Spielman JL. Voice harmonic amplitude differences before and after LSVT LOUD™ in Parkinson's disease. Mov Disord. 2016;31(Suppl 2):S626.
28. Vernier LS, Ramos NC, Cassol M, Marchand DLP. Lee Silverman voice treatment in Parkinson's disease: a systematic review of clinical trials. Int Arch Otorhinolaryngol. 2016;20(Suppl 1):S17.
29. Neves MRL, Brendim MP, Carvalho YSV, Dias Marques CH, Da Silva VG. Immediate effect of semi-occluded vocal tract exercise (high resistance tube) in Parkinson's disease. Int Arch Otorhinolaryngol. 2016;20(Suppl 1):S101.

30. Novotný M, Rusz J, Čmejla R, Růžičková H, Klempíř J, Růžička E. Hypernasality associated with basal ganglia dysfunction: evidence from Parkinson's disease and Huntington's disease. PeerJ. 2016;4:e2530. https://doi.org/10.7717/peerj.2530.
31. Majdinasab F, Karkheiran S, Soltani M, Moradi N, Shahidi G. Relationship between voice and motor disabilities of Parkinson's disease. J Voice. 2016;30(6):768.e17–22. https://doi.org/10.1016/j.jvoice.2015.10.022.
32. Roubeau B, Bruel M, de Crouy CO, Périé S. Reduction of Parkinson's-related dysphonia by thyroplasty. Eur Ann Otorhinolaryngol Head Neck Dis. 2016;133(6):437–9. https://doi.org/10.1016/j.anorl.2016.07.005.
33. Sidtis D, Sidtis JJ. Subcortical effects on voice and fluency in dysarthria: observations from subthalamic nucleus stimulation. J Alzheimers Dis Parkinsonism. 2017;7(6):392. https://doi.org/10.4172/2161-0460.1000392.
34. Wu Y, Chen P, Yao Y, Ye X, Xiao Y, Liao L, et al. Dysphonic voice pattern analysis of patients in Parkinson's disease using minimum interclass probability risk feature selection and bagging ensemble learning methods. Comput Math Methods Med. 2017;2017:4201984. https://doi.org/10.1155/2017/4201984.
35. Stegemöller EL, Radig H, Hibbing P, Wingate J, Sapienza C. Effects of singing on voice, respiratory control, and quality of life in persons with Parkinson's disease. Disabil Rehabil. 2017;39(6):594–600. https://doi.org/10.3109/09638288.2016.1152610.
36. Parveen S, Goberman AM. Comparison of self and proxy ratings for voice handicap index and motor-related quality of life of individuals with Parkinson's disease. Int J Speech Lang Pathol. 2017;19(2):174–83. https://doi.org/10.3109/17549507.2016.1167242.
37. Butala A, Swaminathan A, Dunlop S, Salnikova Y, Ficek B, Portnoff B, et al. Parkinsonics – a prospective, randomized, blinded, cross-over trial of group singing for motor and non-motor symptoms in idiopathic Parkinson's disease (PD). Mov Disord. 2017;32(Suppl 2):457. https://doi.org/10.1002/mds.27087. Abstract 1190
38. Da Silva VG, Dias Marques CH, Neves MRL, Da Veiga TC. Immediate effect of expiratory strengthening training in swallowing and voice in patients with Parkinson's disease. Int Arch Otorhinolaryngol. 2017;21(Suppl 2):S88.
39. Kacha A, Mertens C, Grenez F, Skodda S, Schoentgen J. On the harmonic-to-noise ratio as an acoustic cue of vocal timbre of Parkinson speakers. Biomed Signal Process Control. 2017;37:32–8. https://doi.org/10.1016/j.bspc.2016.09.004.
40. Lechien JR, Blecic S, Ghosez Y, Huet K, Harmegnies B, Saussez S. Voice quality and orofacial strength as outcome of levodopa effectiveness in patients with early idiopathic Parkinson disease: a preliminary report. J Voice. 2019;33(5):716–20. https://doi.org/10.1016/j.jvoice.2018.04.002.
41. Abur D, Lester-Smith RA, Daliri A, Lupiani AA, Guenther FH, Stepp CE. Sensorimotor adaptation of voice fundamental frequency in Parkinson's disease. PLoS One. 2018;13(1):e0191839. https://doi.org/10.1371/journal.pone.0191839.
42. Vieira M, De Resende H, Quintas V, Attoni T, Baracho L, Britto AT, et al. Interaction between vowel lengthening and tonal alignment in Parkinson's disease. Mov Disord. 2018;33(Suppl 2):49–50. https://doi.org/10.1002/mds.27434.
43. Motta S, Cesari U, Paternoster M, Motta G, Orefice G. Aerodynamic findings and voice handicap index in Parkinson's disease. Eur Arch Otorrinolaringol. 2018;275(6):1569–77. https://doi.org/10.1007/s00405-018-4967-7.
44. Lechien JR, Blecic S, Huet K, Delvaux V, Piccaluga M, Roland V, et al. Voice quality outcomes of idiopathic Parkinson's disease medical treatment: a systematic review. Clin Otolaryngol. 2018;43(6):882–903. https://doi.org/10.1111/coa.13082.
45. Abur D, Lupiani AA, Hickox AE, Shinn-Cunningham BG, Stepp CE. Loudness perception of pure tones in Parkinson's disease. J Speech Lang Hear Res. 2018;61(6):1487–96. https://doi.org/10.1044/2018_JSLHR-H-17-0382.
46. Ko EJ, Chae M, Cho SR. Relationship between swallowing function and maximum phonation time in patients with parkinsonism. Ann Rehabil Med. 2018;42(3):425–32. https://doi.org/10.5535/arm.2018.42.3.425.

47. Han EY, Yun JY, Chong HJ, Choi KG. Individual therapeutic singing program for vocal quality and depression in Parkinson's disease. J Mov Disord. 2018;11(3):121–8. https://doi.org/10.14802/jmd.17078.
48. Manor Y, Naor S, Shpunt D, Diamant N, Zivion N, Hayat L, et al. Acoustic analysis and subjective vocal perception of Parkinson's disease patients and healthy control and the relation to depression and quality of life [abstract]. Mov Disord. 2018;33(Suppl 2)
49. Pinho P, Monteiro L, Soares MFP, Tourinho L, Melo A, Nóbrega AC. Impact of levodopa treatment in the voice pattern of Parkinson's disease patients: a systematic review and meta-analysis. Codas. 2018;30(5):e20170200. https://doi.org/10.1590/2317-1782/20182017200.
50. Gillivan-Murphy P, Miller N, Carding P. Voice tremor in Parkinson's disease: an acoustic study. J Voice. 2019;33(4):526–35. https://doi.org/10.1016/j.jvoice.2017.12.010.
51. Shen J, Zhang T, Huang F, Zhou H, Teng F, Kim H, Jin L. Study of voice disorder based on acoustic assessment in Parkinson's disease. Chin J Neurol. 2019;52(8):613–9. https://doi.org/10.3760/cma.j.issn.1006-7876.2019.08.003.
52. Saffarian A, Amiri Shavaki Y, Shahidi GA, Hadavi S, Jafari Z. Lee Silverman voice treatment (LSVT) mitigates voice difficulties in mild Parkinson's disease. Med J Islam Repub Iran. 2019 Jan;30(33):5. https://doi.org/10.34171/mjiri.33.5.
53. Romann AJ, Beber BC, Cielo CA, Rieder CRM. Acoustic voice modifications in individuals with Parkinson disease submitted to deep brain stimulation. Int Arch Otorhinolaryngol. 2019;23(2):203–8. https://doi.org/10.1055/s-0038-1675392.
54. Arora S, Baghai-Ravary L, Tsanas A. Developing a large scale population screening tool for the assessment of Parkinson's disease using telephone-quality voice. J Acoust Soc Am. 2019;145(5):2871. https://doi.org/10.1121/1.5100272.
55. Behroozmand R, Johari K, Kelley RM, Kapnoula EC, Narayanan NS, Greenlee JDW. Effect of deep brain stimulation on vocal motor control mechanisms in Parkinson's disease. Parkinsonism Relat Disord. 2019;63:46–53. https://doi.org/10.1016/j.parkreldis.2019.03.002.
56. Finger ME, Madden LL, Haq IU, McLouth CJ, Siddiqui MS. Analysis of the prevalence and onset of dysphonia and dysphagia symptoms in movement disorders at an academic medical center. J Clin Neurosci. 2019;64:111–5. https://doi.org/10.1016/j.jocn.2019.03.043.
57. Karlsson F, Malinova E, Olofsson K, Blomstedt P, Linder J, Nordh E. Voice tremor outcomes of subthalamic nucleus and zona incerta deep brain stimulation in patients with Parkinson disease. J Voice. 2019;33(4):545–9. https://doi.org/10.1016/j.jvoice.2017.12.012.
58. Sheibani R, Nikookar E, Alavi SE. An ensemble method for diagnosis of Parkinson's disease based on voice measurements. J Med Signals Sens. 2019;9(4):221–6. https://doi.org/10.4103/jmss.JMSS_57_18.
59. Tamplin J, Morris ME, Marigliani C, Baker FA, Noffs G, Vogel AP. ParkinSong: outcomes of a 12-month controlled trial of therapeutic singing groups in Parkinson's disease. J Parkinsons Dis. 2020;10(3):1217–30. https://doi.org/10.3233/JPD-191838.
60. Viswanathan R, Arjunan SP, Bingham A, Jelfs B, Kempster P, Raghav S, Kumar DK. Complexity measures of voice recordings as a discriminative tool for Parkinson's disease. Biosensors (Basel). 2020;10(1):1. https://doi.org/10.3390/bios10010001.
61. Nakayama K, Yamamoto T, Oda C, Sato M, Murakami T, Horiguchi S. Effectiveness of Lee Silverman Voice Treatment® LOUD on Japanese-speaking patients with Parkinson's disease. Rehabil Res Pract. 2020;2020:6585264. https://doi.org/10.1155/2020/6585264.
62. Ma A, Lau KK, Thyagarajan D. Voice changes in Parkinson's disease: what are they telling us? J Clin Neurosci. 2020;72:1–7. https://doi.org/10.1016/j.jocn.2019.12.029.
63. Morello ANDC, Beber BC, Fagundes VC, Cielo CA, Rieder CRM. Dysphonia and dysarthria in people with Parkinson's disease after subthalamic nucleus deep brain stimulation: effect of frequency modulation. J Voice. 2020;34(3):477–84. https://doi.org/10.1016/j.jvoice.2018.10.012.
64. Chiaramonte R, Bonfiglio M. Acoustic analysis of voice in Parkinson's disease: a systematic review of voice disability and meta-analysis of studies. Rev Neurol. 2020;70(11):393–405. https://doi.org/10.33588/rn.7011.2019414.

65. Viswanathan R, Arjunan SP, Kempster P, Raghav S, Kumar DK. Estimation of Parkinson's disease severity from voice features of vowels and consonant. In: Proceedings of the 42nd annual international conference of the IEEE Engineering in Medicine and Biology Society (EMBC); 2020. p. 3666–9. https://doi.org/10.1109/EMBC44109.2020.9175395.
66. Altay EV, Alatas B. Association analysis of Parkinson disease with vocal change characteristics using multi-objective metaheuristic optimization. Med Hypotheses. 2020;141:109722. https://doi.org/10.1016/j.mehy.2020.109722.
67. Park JE, Oh SW, Shin JY, Lee SY, Hong SH, Ahn NH, et al. (Say "AH~"): Vocal Analysis in Parkinson's Disease and Essential Tremor [abstract]. Mov Disord. 2020;35(suppl 1)
68. Sarac ET, Yilmaz A, Aydinli FE, Yildizgoren MT, Okuyucu EE, Okuyucu S, Akakin A. Investigating the effects of subthalamic nucleus-deep brain stimulation on the voice quality. Somatosens Mot Res. 2020;37(3):157–64. https://doi.org/10.1080/08990220.2020.1761317.
69. Reyes A, Castillo A, Castillo J, Cornejo I, Cruickshank T. The effects of respiratory muscle training on phonatory measures in individuals with Parkinson's disease. J Voice. 2019;34(6):894–902. https://doi.org/10.1016/j.jvoice.2019.05.001.
70. Lechien JR, Delsaut B, Abderrakib A, Huet K, Delvaux V, Piccaluga M, et al. Orofacial strength and voice quality as outcome of levodopa challenge test in Parkinson disease. Laryngoscope. 2020;130(12):E896–903. https://doi.org/10.1002/lary.28645.
71. Gaballah A, Parsa V, Andreetta M, Adams S. Assessment of amplified Parkinsonian speech quality using deep learning. In: IEEE Canadian Conference on Electrical & Computer Engineering (CCECE), vol. 2018. Quebec: IEEE; 2018. p. 1–4. https://doi.org/10.1109/CCECE.2018.8447721.
72. Lechien JR, Huet K, Finck C, Blecic S, Delvaux V, Piccaluga M, et al. Are the acoustic measurements reliable in the assessment of voice quality? A methodological prospective study. J Voice. 2021;35(2):203–15. https://doi.org/10.1016/j.jvoice.2019.08.022.
73. Jain A, Abedinpour K, Polat O, Çalışkan MM, Asaei A, Pfister FMJ, et al. Voice analysis to differentiate the dopaminergic response in people with Parkinson's disease. Front Hum Neurosci. 2021;15:667997. https://doi.org/10.3389/fnhum.2021.667997.
74. Gaballah A, Parsa V, Cushnie-Sparrow D, Adams S. Improved estimation of parkinsonian vowel quality through acoustic feature assimilation. Sci World J. 2021;2021:6076828. https://doi.org/10.1155/2021/6076828.
75. Rajasekar SJS, Narayanan V, Perumal V. ParkAI – an AI based tool for detection of Parkinson's disease using vocal measurements. Mov Disord. 2021;36(suppl 1):1.
76. Da Silva JMS, Gomes AOC, Da Silva HJ, De Vasconcelos SJ, De Sales Coriolano MDW, De Lira ZS. Effect of resonance tube technique on oropharyngeal geometry and voice in individuals with Parkinson's disease. J Voice. 2021;35(5):807.e25–32. https://doi.org/10.1016/j.jvoice.2020.01.025.
77. Searl J, Dietsch AM. Daily Phonatory activity of individuals with Parkinson's disease. J Voice. 2024;38(3):800.e13–26. https://doi.org/10.1016/j.jvoice.2021.10.004.
78. Koyuncu H, Fidan V, Toktas H, Binay O, Celik H. Effect of ketogenic diet versus regular diet on voice quality of patients with Parkinson's disease. Acta Neurol Belg. 2021;121(6):1729–32. https://doi.org/10.1007/s13760-020-01486-0.
79. Yasar OC, Ozturk S, Kemal O, Kocabicak E. Effects of subthalamic nucleus deep brain stimulation surgery on voice and formant frequencies of vowels in Turkish. Turk Neurosurg. 2022;32(5):764–72. https://doi.org/10.5137/1019-5149.JTN.36134-21.2.
80. Rajeswari SS, Nair M. Prediction of Parkinson's disease from voice signals using machine learning. J Pharm Negat Results. 2022;13(S7):294. https://doi.org/10.47750/pnr.2022.13.S07.294.
81. Suppa A, Costantini G, Asci F, Di Leo P, Al-Wardat MS, Di Lazzaro G, et al. Voice in Parkinson's disease: a machine learning study. Front Neurol. 2022;13:831428. https://doi.org/10.3389/fneur.2022.831428.

82. Yu Q, Zou X, Quan F, Dong Z, Yin H, Liu J, et al. Parkinson's disease patients with freezing of gait have more severe voice impairment than non-freezers during "ON State". J Neural Transm (Vienna). 2022;129(3):277–86. https://doi.org/10.1007/s00702-021-02458-1.
83. Paulino CEB, Silva HJD, Gomes AOC, Silva JMSD, Cunha DAD, Coriolano MDGWS, et al. Relationship between oropharyngeal geometry and vocal parameters in subjects with Parkinson's disease. J Voice. 2022;S0892-1997(22):00021–2. https://doi.org/10.1016/j.jvoice.2022.01.020.
84. Kopf LM, Rohl AHG, Nagao T, Bryant KNT, Johari K, Tjaden K, et al. Voice handicap index in Parkinson's patients: subthalamic versus Globus Pallidus deep brain stimulation. J Clin Neurosci. 2022;98:83–8. https://doi.org/10.1016/j.jocn.2022.01.029.
85. Vojtech JM, Stepp CE. Effects of age and Parkinson's disease on the relationship between vocal fold abductory kinematics and relative fundamental frequency. J Voice. 2022;S0892-1997(22):00070–4. https://doi.org/10.1016/j.jvoice.2022.03.007.
86. Dos Santos AP, Troche MS, Berretin-Felix G, Barbieri FA, Brasolotto AG, Silverio KCA. Effects of resonance tube voice therapy on Parkinson's disease: clinical trial. J Voice. 2022;S0892-1997(22):00126–6. https://doi.org/10.1016/j.jvoice.2022.04.016.
87. Pah ND, Motin MA, Kumar DK. Phonemes based detection of Parkinson's disease for telehealth applications. Sci Rep. 2022;12:10412. https://doi.org/10.1038/s41598-022-13865-z.
88. Bao G, Lin M, Sang X, Hou Y, Liu Y, Wu Y. Classification of dysphonic voices in Parkinson's disease with semi-supervised competitive learning algorithm. Biosensors. 2022;12(7):502. https://doi.org/10.3390/bios12070502.
89. Marchese MR, Proietti I, Longobardi Y, Mari G, Cefaro CA, D'Alatri L. Multidimensional voice assessment after Lee Silverman voice therapy (LSVT®) in Parkinson's disease. Acta Otorhinolaryngol Ital. 2022;42(4):348–54. https://doi.org/10.14639/0392-100X-N1962.
90. Dao SVT, Yu Z, Tran LV, Phan PNK, Huynh TTM, Le TM. An analysis of vocal features for Parkinson's disease classification using evolutionary algorithms. Diagnostics (Basel). 2022;12(8):1980. https://doi.org/10.3390/diagnostics12081980.
91. Atalar MS, Genç G, Oğur Ş. Comparison of voice, speech, swallowing, and drooling problems in Parkinson's disease patients with healthy individuals [abstract]. Mov Disord. 2022;37(suppl 2) Available from: https://www.mdsabstracts.org/abstract/comparison-of-voice-speech-swallowing-and-drooling-problems-in-parkinsons-disease-patients-with-healthy-individuals/. Accessed 29 Apr 2024
92. Butala A, Li K, Swaminathan A, Dunlop S, Salnikova Y, Ficek B, et al. Parkinsonics: a randomized, blinded, cross-over trial of group singing for motor and nonmotor symptoms in idiopathic Parkinson disease. Parkinsons Dis. 2022;2022:4233203. https://doi.org/10.1155/2022/4233203.
93. Lim WS, Chiu S, Wu M, Tsai S, Wang P, Lin K, et al. An integrated biometric voice and facial features for early detection of Parkinson's disease. NPJ Parkinsons Dis. 2022;8(1):145. https://doi.org/10.1038/s41531-022-00414-8.
94. Good A, Earle E, Vezer E, Gilmore S, Livingstone S, Russo FA. Community choir improves vocal production measures in individuals living with Parkinson's disease. J Voice. 2023;37(2):203–14. https://doi.org/10.1016/j.jvoice.2022.12.001.
95. Cabestany J, Suppa A, ÓLaighin G. Editorial: Parkinson's disease: technological trends for diagnosis and treatment improvement. Front Neurol. 2023;14:1151858. https://doi.org/10.3389/fneur.2023.1151858.
96. Costantini G, Cesarini V, Di Leo P, Amato F, Suppa A, Asci F, et al. Artificial intelligence-based voice assessment of patients with Parkinson's disease off and on treatment: machine vs. deep-learning comparison. Sensors (Basel). 2023;23(4):2293. https://doi.org/10.3390/s23042293.
97. Li Q, Millard K, Tetnowski J, Narayana S, Cannito M. Acoustic analysis of intonation in persons with Parkinson's disease receiving transcranial magnetic stimulation and intensive voice treatment. J Voice. 2023;37(2):203–14. https://doi.org/10.1016/j.jvoice.2020.12.019.

98. Olivares A, Comini L, Di Pietro DA, Vezzadini G, Luisa A, Boccali E, et al. Perceptual and qualitative voice alterations detected by GIRBAS in patients with Parkinson's disease: is there a relation with lung function and oxygenation? Aging Clin Exp Res. 2023;35(3):633–8. https://doi.org/10.1007/s40520-022-02324-4.
99. Silva JMSD, Gomes AOC, Coriolano MDGWS, Teixeira JP, Lima HVSL, Paulino CEB, Silva HJD, Lira ZS. Oropharyngeal geometry and acoustic parameters of voice in healthy and Parkinson's disease subjects. CoDAS. 2023;35(2):e20210304. https://doi.org/10.1590/2317-1782/20232021304pt.
100. Abraham EA, Geetha A. Acoustical and perceptual analysis of voice in individuals with Parkinson's disease. Indian J Otolaryngol Head Neck Surg. 2023;75(2):427–32. https://doi.org/10.1007/s12070-022-03282-z.
101. Lima HVSL, Lopes LW, Silva HJD, Vieira ACC, Cruz TVSD, Gomes AOC, Lira ZS. Performance of the phonatory deviation diagram in monitoring voice quality before and after voice exercise in individuals with Parkinson's disease. CoDAS. 2023;35(4):e20210224. https://doi.org/10.1590/2317-1782/20232021224pt.
102. Manor Y, Kochetkov Y, Hauptman Y, Shpunt D, Zait A, Gurevich T. Analysis of the relationship between acoustic measures and VHI score [abstract]. Mov Disord. 2023;38(suppl 1)
103. Romero Arias T, Redondo Cortés I, Pérez Del Olmo A. Biomechanical parameters of voice in Parkinson's disease patients. Folia Phoniatr Logop. 2024;76(1):91–101. https://doi.org/10.1159/000533289.
104. Pedersen M. Artificial intelligence for screening voice disorders: aspects of risk factors: research article. Am J Med Clin Res Rev. 2025;4(2):1–8. https://doi.org/10.58372/2835-6276.1254.
105. Ngo QC, Motin MA, Pah ND, Drotár P, Kempster P, Kumar D. Computerized analysis of speech and voice for Parkinson's disease: a systematic review. Comput Methods Prog Biomed. 2022;226:107133. https://doi.org/10.1016/j.cmpb.2022.107133.
106. Idrisoglu A, Dallora AL, Anderberg P, Berglund JS. Applied machine learning techniques to diagnose voice-affecting conditions and disorders: systematic literature review. J Med Internet Res. 2023;25:e46105. https://doi.org/10.2196/46105.

Open Access This chapter is licensed under the terms of the Creative Commons Attribution-NonCommercial-NoDerivatives 4.0 International License (http://creativecommons.org/licenses/by-nc-nd/4.0/), which permits any noncommercial use, sharing, distribution and reproduction in any medium or format, as long as you give appropriate credit to the original author(s) and the source, provide a link to the Creative Commons license and indicate if you modified the licensed material. You do not have permission under this license to share adapted material derived from this chapter or parts of it.

The images or other third party material in this chapter are included in the chapter's Creative Commons license, unless indicated otherwise in a credit line to the material. If material is not included in the chapter's Creative Commons license and your intended use is not permitted by statutory regulation or exceeds the permitted use, you will need to obtain permission directly from the copyright holder.

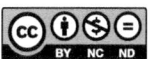

AI-Enhanced Voice Analysis for Neurological Diseases

Neveen Hassan Nashaat

3.1 Introduction

The number of adults with neurological disorders is rising worldwide. Neurological disorders are considered the leading cause of disability or ill health worldwide [1]. Early diagnosis of these disorders, especially neurodegenerative disorders, is essential for proper management and reducing complications and rapid progress. Although these disorders influence different body systems, changes in voice (dysphonia) usually appear before other symptoms. The use of artificial intelligence (AI) and machine learning for early diagnosis of voice pathology in neurological disorders is a rapidly emerging research field, and it is seen as particularly promising [2]. Previous research studies tried to quantify neurological disorders using different modalities to obtain a holistic and longitudinal picture of a patient, identify the course of the neurological disorder, and, favorably, its early detection. Voice recordings are readily available and unobtrusive due to the widespread use of smartphones, making their use convenient for neurological disorders [3].

When a speech sample is obtained to be processed by AI, it undergoes quality enhancement through dereverberation and denoising. Then, analysis of data is performed by processing the data, followed by applying analytical methods for feature extraction. These features stemming from the acoustic aspects of the recorded speech signal are used to quantify voice measures. Generally, there are several approaches to the analysis of data. They include statistical analysis, predictive modeling, and artificial neural networks. Statistical methods are used to detect significant correlations of individual features for the targeted disorder. The determined correlated features could represent the voice biomarkers of a disorder. In predictive modeling, machine learning is used to build statistical models for recognizing

N. H. Nashaat (✉)
Research on Children with Special Needs Department, Medical Research and Clinical Studies Institute, National Research Centre, Cairo, Egypt

© The Author(s) 2026
M. Pedersen et al. (eds.), *Voice-related Biomarkers*,
https://doi.org/10.1007/978-3-032-03134-1_3

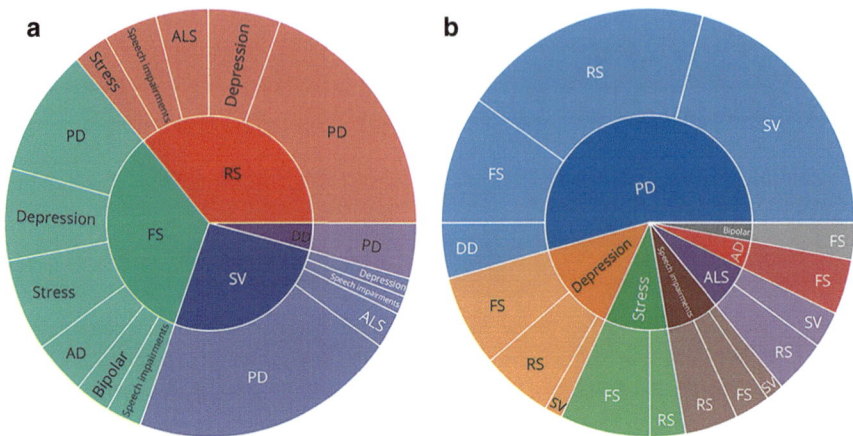

Fig. 3.1 Proportion of neurological disorders and speech tasks. Charts representing the proportion of neurological disorders and speech tasks analyzed by AI in previous studies (**a**) speech tasks in the inner circle, (**b**) disorders in the inner circle. *AD* Alzheimer's disease, *ALS* amyotrophic lateral sclerosis, *DD* diadochokinesis, *FS* free speech, *PD* Parkinson's disease, *RS* read speech, *SV* sustained vowels. (Copyright: Hecker P, Steckhan N, Eyben F, Schuller BW, and Arnrich B (2022) [3], redistributed under the terms of the Creative Commons Attribution License (CC BY))

categories specific to a certain disorder. Artificial neural networks could be used when plenty of data is available [4].

Alzheimer's disease, amyotrophic lateral sclerosis, and Parkinson's disease (PD) are the main neurological disorders targeted by AI using extracted voice and speech data. Some of these disorders and the samples used for analysis using AI are presented in Fig. 3.1. Recently, the automated speech recognition system enabled automatic transcription of speech content, such as silent pauses, articulation rate, and hesitation ratio in the recorded speech [5]. Smartphone technology has expanded diagnostic capabilities, enabling the assessment of symptoms in dexterity and gait [6]. There has been research showing that AI-enhanced acoustic voice measurements are accurate in distinguishing between patients and healthy controls, with high classification and staging accuracy in many studies. Multi-classifier frameworks, autonomous feature extraction systems, and ensemble learning, for example, have been employed to improve PD classification accuracy [7].

There is heterogeneity and variability in the types of evaluation when considering the software that has been used for the analysis, the type of statistical analysis, and the algorithm used. Therefore, there are issues in this field, and this chapter will mostly focus on the current challenges and how to find solutions to them.

3.2 Perspectives

3.2.1 The Use of AI in the Detection of Voice Pathology of Neurological Disorders

AI can analyze large volumes of data, explore possible biomarkers, and improve management accuracy. One of the AI tools is machine learning. Its algorithms can process extensive sets of data and patients' information. Consequently, accurate models for diagnosis, treatment, and prediction are developed. When an algorithm encodes some statistical regularities inherent in a database of examples into parameter weights for certain future predictions, that is called machine learning. Deep learning (DL) is a subcategory of machine learning. The difference between them is how much data each type uses and how each one learns. DL enables the use of large data sets [8]. Besides traditional machine learning and DL, model-based transfer learning (model-TL) is used to transfer the knowledge that is learned from the source domain into the target one. For example, the deep convolutional neural network (CNN) classifier, which is based on the model-TL, was used to recognize patients with Parkinson's disease utilizing voice biomarkers extracted from sustained vowels [9].

3.2.2 Computerized Tools Used for Voice and Speech Analysis

Several procedures were created to assess neurological disorders via voice and speech analysis. To extract features, PRAAT, VOICEBOX, and OPENSMILE (open-source Speech and Music Interpretation by Large-space Extraction) toolkits could be used. The bag-of-audio-words (BOAWS) could be elicited using the OPENXBOW framework for the recognition of emotions from speech [3]. Testing speed and fluency of speech could also be performed using PRAAT software to extract voiced and unvoiced parts of a sound signal. It measures the time, frequency, duration, and quality of the signals [10]. The brightness of a sound is measured by the spectral centroid, which is the acoustic descriptor of timbre [11]. Voice and acoustic characteristics include noise-to-harmonic ratio, pitch, intensity, and other measures. The "Duration Characteristics" quantify the voice breaks and unvoiced frames. The prosody and paralinguistic feature sets obtained from a temporal domain of the speech signal are measured by Emotional Temperature Analysis [11].

3.2.3 Voice and Speech Analysis by AI

In the field of disease recognition from voice measures, machine learning methods including CNNs, Random Forests (RF), Long Short-Term Memory (LSTM) networks, Feed Forward Neural Networks, k-nearest Neighbors (KNN), and Regression Trees (RT) were commonly used. CNNs learn directly from the raw audio waveform or from feature representations of spectrograms of audio signals. They contain either architectural elements to perform a classification decision within the network architecture, or other predictive modeling approaches are employed based on these feature representations [12]. For a successful use of AI for voice analysis, the fidelity of the recorded speech should be sufficient, the accuracy of the analytical algorithm used for analysis should be guaranteed, and the repeatability of the measures should be ensured [13]. In neurological disorders, voice and speech impairments occur at various phases, demonstrating their importance in distinguishing the stages and forecasting their progression [14]. The AuDEEP algorithm utilizes spectrograms from the audio signals input to train the encoder-decoder networks without providing a sequence-to-sequence autoencoder (class labels) specific to the targeted data. Then, the outputs of the trained encoder could be utilized to output features as abstract representations based on the input signal spectrograms [15].

3.2.4 AI-Enhanced Voice Analysis in Alzheimer's Disease

Alzheimer's disease (AD) is a type of dementia that affects the memory, cognition, and motor abilities of patients. Acoustic and other features revealed information indicative of AD. These features include paralinguistic, prosodic, and non-verbal features such as the amount of silence [16]. Acoustic and linguistic measures could be augmented with verbal memory scoring to further improve AD detection. The verbal memory tasks could be automatically scored utilizing technologies for natural language processing. Integrating the acoustic and linguistic features was reported to achieve an accuracy of more than 85% for distinguishing patients positive for beta-amyloid from others, in addition to recognizing patients with mild cognitive impairment [17]. The acoustic voice measures used included jitter, shimmer, pitch, intensity, the Hammarberg index, the alpha ratio, the frequency of some formants, cepstral parameters, and relative energy. Furthermore, frequency analysis, such as variance, mean, and kurtosis of Mel-frequency cepstral coefficients (MFCC), could be utilized. The phonation rate, pause rate, and periodicity of speech, representing temporal analysis, could aid in the analysis [18]. The datasets that have been used varied across studies and were sometimes imbalanced. The limitations made it challenging to compare the efficacy of different modalities. However, this field is considered a promising research topic.

Large Language Models (LLMs) or machine learning methods such as the Bidirectional Encoder Representations from Transformers (BERT) and Generative Pre-trained Transformer 3 were previously used for AD patients in Agbavor and Liang's study [18]. Classifying AD could be performed utilizing a fully connected three-layer feedforward neural network (NN) with a sigmoid function as a final layer. This has led to originating a score for AD. Obtaining a score of 0.5 or more suggested having AD, whereas a score less than 0.5 indicated a non-AD condition. For AD severity estimation, a regression model using a neural network composed of an input layer, two hidden layers, and an output layer has been utilized. The cognitive test (Mini-Mental State Examination) was used to achieve this goal. The scores obtained for grading suggested the 20–24 score to categorize mild dementia, the 13 to 20 score for moderate degree, and less than 12 for severe dementia. The data2vec, which is a general framework for self-supervised learning, was reported to be better than the wav2vec2 algorithm method for voice measures recognizing AD [18].

3.2.5 AI-Enhanced Voice Analysis in Amyotrophic Lateral Sclerosis

Amyotrophic lateral sclerosis is a neurodegenerative disorder causing deficits in motor control and cognitive performance, in addition to lower motor neuron lesions influencing speech and voice. Measures such as shimmer, jitter, fundamental frequency (F0), harmonic-to-noise ratio (HNR), loudness, pause duration, and zero-crossings were used to categorize patients from healthy controls aided by AI. Classification was accomplished using a Bayesian LASSO (Least Absolute Shrinkage and Selection Operator) logistic regression model [19]. Speaking intensity, speaking rate, and F0 distributional characteristics, especially the standard deviation of F0 and shimmer, revealed having higher weights than other voice and speech measures [20]. F0 range and maximum F0 were useful for predicting intelligibility reduction [21]. The intensity features were related to respiratory muscle weakness. For staging, the Winterlight pipeline could stratify patients into the early stage and late bulbar stage [19].

3.2.6 AI-Enhanced Voice Analysis in Multiple Sclerosis

Multiple sclerosis (MS) is a chronic autoimmune disorder affecting the central nervous system, creating inflammatory plaques that cause demyelination and axonal transection. The RF model performed well, achieving high accuracy for validation and training targeting this disorder [22]. Gosztolya and Egas-López [23] utilized Wav2vec 2.0 models and the cross-lingual models and found the latter better in discrimination.

Voice analysis features and the vowel space area (VSA) using the K-NN were successful in discriminating patients with MS from controls (95%). VSA was utilized to quantify the quadrilateral extent formed when the vowels at the four corners are projected in the initial Formant 1 (F1) and Formant 2 (F2). It is calculated to judge the articulation and the centralization of vocal sounds. It reflects the modifications of speech motor control. High VSA represents healthy speech or hyperarticulated sounds, whereas low VSA results from pathological conditions [24].

3.2.7 AI-Enhanced Voice Analysis in Mild Cognitive Impairment

Mild Cognitive Impairment (MCI) is considered a predementia stage. It is expected that one in five people aged 65 years or older will develop dementia by 2025. It is difficult to distinguish MCI from other disorders, such as the early stages of depression. Thus, voice analysis has been proposed. Telephonic speech samples were used to collect voice and speech features related to silence intervals, prosody, intensity of voice, and pitch. The obtained accuracy for MCI detection was 90% [25]. When logistic regression was used for many voice features obtained by openSMILE and INTERSPEECH, such as F0, fast Fourier transform (FFT), voiced sound probability, MFCC, energy, and zero-crossing rate, the area under the curve (AUC) was high (0.9) [26].

3.2.8 AI-Enhanced Voice Analysis in Ataxia

Ataxia is the loss of motor coordination. Cerebellar ataxia results in ataxic dysarthria. Acoustic features concerning spectrum, time, cepstral, and non-linear dynamics obtained from the repetition of different consonant-vowel syllable paradigms obtained by a microphone revealed a balanced accuracy of 91.2% for ataxia recognition [27]. A neural network, which was trained for phoneme prediction, was applied to the t (AVE) was computed for the participant's recording, along with intensity standard deviations and mean pitch in the vowel segments. The data demonstrated the ability to capture the disorder progression [28]. Song et al. [29] developed a patch-wise wave-splitting and integrating AI system for audio classification (PWSI-AI-AC) to overcome problems related to insufficient data in the medical field for the DL model. CNN's model for waveform was used to differentiate between hypokinetic and ataxic speech. The AUC performance was up to 0.9 with an accuracy of 80%.

3.2.9 AI-Enhanced Voice Analysis in Wilson's Disease

Wilson's disease (WD) is attributed to ATP7B gene variation leading to the accumulation of copper in the brain and liver. It has variable patterns and outcomes. Using voice analysis of sustained vowels was proposed for WD identification by Zhang et al. [30], who utilized the improved MFCC using signal decomposition. The classification accuracy achieved was 86.1%. Zhang et al. [31] utilized the bidirectional LSTM network with an attention mechanism for analyzing unstructured connected speech. A duration of about 30 seconds was sufficient for recognizing WD. The Mel spectrograms revealed short utterances, slow, laborious articulation, and disorganized rhythms [31].

3.2.10 AI-Enhanced Voice Analysis in Essential Voice Tremor

Essential voice tremor (EVT) is a form of discoordination within the laryngeal musculature. It leads to fluctuations at a low frequency of the F0 and reduced strength of the excitation amplitude. Support Vector Machine (SVM) was used as a classifier for EVT using pitch contour [32]. Moreover, the power spectral analysis of sustained vowels and SVM helped in the objective detection of EVT [33].

3.2.11 AI-Enhanced Voice Analysis in Huntington's Disease

Huntington's disease (HD) is a dominant autosomal neurodegenerative disorder resulting from the mutant huntingtin gene (HTT), resulting in premature brain atrophy and neuronal dysfunctions. Inappropriate silences, mono-pitch, imprecision of consonants, variable rates, and dysphonic voice are distinctive characteristics of the hyperkinetic dysarthria associated with chorea [34]. The voice and speech features were reported to be valuable digital measures of HD detection and progression. Extracting pitch, accuracy, and pausing was performed from counting forward, counting backward, and completing passage reading. RF machine learning models were utilized for clinical status determination and for disease severity and progression judgment, making these models promising for their remote and frequent assessment [35]. Other speech features were used for AI analysis for HD discrimination from healthy controls using dynamic features and static ones. Goodness of pronunciation, speech rate, pauses, and speech fillers (um, uh, etc.) were used. The k-NN and LSTM were used for the dynamic features. The k-NN and DNN modeled the static features [36].

3.2.12 AI-Enhanced Voice Analysis in Parkinson's Disease

Parkinson's Disease (PD) is a neurodegenerative disorder characterized by the loss of neurons producing dopamine in the substantia nigra [37]. Large-scale studies, such as the Parkinson's Speech Initiative, aim to distinguish PD patients from controls using phone-quality voice in non-acoustically controlled environments. Triggering the articulatory and voice deficits in PD was more efficient in monologs than in other speech tasks, such as structured speech tasks during picture description [38].

DL is increasingly used for processing complex voice signal issues in PD research. Ensemble methods, CNNs, SVMs, RFs, decision trees, artificial neural networks, KNNs, multi-layer perceptrons, classification and regression trees, and other machine learning techniques have achieved high accuracy in detecting and staging PD from speech samples. Privacy-sensitive methods for classifying PD have been developed, utilizing passively recorded voice calls and language-aware training of classifiers. The process involves converting speech signals into feature tensors or vectors for DL models, taking into account variations due to the speaker's native language. Multiple DL architectures, like 1D CNN models, have been tested to detect PD with nearly 87% accuracy. Sparse Kernel Transfer Learning was proposed with an accuracy of 86.7%. Deep dual-side learning models with weighted fusion mechanisms achieved higher accuracy, reaching 98.4%. Traditional CNNs have been utilized on the Max Little dataset with an accuracy of 93.10%. SVM with recursive feature elimination utilized a few vocal features necessary to diagnose Parkinson's, with 93.84% accuracy attained [7].

3.2.13 AI-Enhanced Voice Analysis in Depression

Depression is a neuropsychiatric disorder leading to impaired emotional regulation, impaired concentration, and reduced interest, in addition to suicidal contemplation. The detection of depression from voice analysis was reported to show good discrimination and grading performance. CNN, Temporal Dilated Convolutional Network, RF, and LSTM were utilized for depression detection. Jitter, MFCC, and glottal flow spectrum were found to be associated with the severity of depression. The wav2vec 2.0 pre-training model for voice was used to extract high-quality voice features from raw audio signals. A large amount of voice data was utilized to train the wav2vec model [39]. Shin et al. [40] used machine learning to differentiate minor depression from major depressive disorder with a specificity of 66.2% and a sensitivity of 65.6%. The glottal closure instance, the opening phase, the closing phase, and the closed phase were obtained through inverse filtering. Formant features, temporal features, and spectral features such as spectral bandwidth, averaged spectral centroid, root mean square energy, and roll-off frequency were extracted. SVM, Gaussian Naive Bayes, logistic regression, and multilayer perceptron were the machine learning algorithms used [40].

3.3 Discussion

The technology for voice analysis has significantly improved over the past ten years due to the advancements in machine learning and DL. However, there are some limitations and challenges regarding the use of AI in voice and speech analysis. Limitations of the current studies using AI for neurological disorder recognition and prognosis in adults include small cohort sizes, which affect the generalizability of results [41]. Gauder et al. [42] suggested collecting datasets under strictly controlled acoustic conditions to avoid the low-accuracy outputs obtained by smartphones, which could further reduce the amount of available data. Nonetheless, recent advances in mobile technology could enable the use of smartphones. Previous studies achieved neurological disease recognition using phone-quality samples with high accuracy [6, 25]. Other challenges include privacy concerns and a lack of standardized datasets. The AI models should have adequate interpretability to enable clinicians to comprehend and trust the results of these models [14]. It has been noticed that the interpretation of some terms differed between studies. For example, Tóth et al. [5] used the term acoustic analysis to describe speech features, such as speech tempo, silent pause, and articulation rate. This interpretation differs from the phoniatricians' perspectives regarding acoustic analysis, which implies voice analysis measures such as F0, HNR, etc.

Recently, feature selection became automatic, and it has improved as transformer utilization has started. This is attributed to different architectures in terms of models in DL, which allow using automatic attention that is applied to the text, image, and voice. These data contribute to developing a foundation model. It is a big model, which is able to manage different types of inputs. The main outcome when using a foundation model is enabling the transformation of the input into embeddings. Embeddings are hyperdimensional vectors that can be represented as a point in a hyperdimensional space. The embedding is located according to the characteristics of the input. The embeddings in the embedding space have the advantage of being the same regardless of the input types. In other words, researchers could transform embeddings from voice, images, or any type of input, which will be introduced directly to the hyperdimensional space in the same way [43]. DL techniques were suggested to improve model performance, including data normalization, feature selection, and avoiding data leakage. Current DL models, which were reported to be used for voice analysis, include CNNs, transformers, autoencoders, recurrent neural networks, and hybrid models, either hybrid DL or hybrid DL models with traditional classifiers [44]. The learned representations of speech signals could be extracted with DEEPSPECTRUM, which uses CNNs [12].

Another challenge is the cross-language classification of neurological disorders. Bertini et al. [45] suggested the use of an end-to-end autoencoder model trained on spectrograms for spontaneous speech to overcome this problem. The main difference between machine learning and DL is that with DL, or even with transformer-based algorithms, feature extraction is not performed. The potential approach would be to collect a data set for pathological and normal voices and perform large-scale, self-supervised learning with DL or transformers. DL techniques help build foundation models for voice. A very large foundation model would enable the researchers to even take into account the differences in different languages and still get an adequate classification even with sentences [46]. An additional solution for improving the AI models is multimodality. Shimoda et al. [25] used speech and voice data to reinforce the detection of dementia. Voice, speech, and cognitive tests were used for AD discrimination [14].

Using AI for voice and speech analysis has many advantages, making it promising for clinical practice. Researchers underscored its importance as a guide in health care systems and telemedicine. Voice can be recorded and monitored over time, which helps reduce anxiety or stress in clinical settings. It is non-invasive, and it is considered cost-effective compared to other investigations, such as magnetic resonance imaging (MRI). Identifying the disorder and its possible grading could aid clinicians in making informed decisions on medication and on other forms of therapy and rehabilitation, which help personalize them, such as phoniatric and physical therapy procedures. Consequently, costs will be reduced, progress will speed up, and clinical trials can be shortened [47].

3.4 Conclusion

The AI-enhanced voice analysis using the DL models presents itself as a cost-effective and non-invasive, promising technology for earlier detection, staging, and progression monitoring of neurological diseases. These models could be applied to voice measures in neurodegenerative disorders, considering that the early detection of these disorders helps reduce the burden on the healthcare systems, improves the quality of life, and prolongs independence.

The high accuracy rates obtained by implementing multimodality, such as linguisic and acoustic features for AD and voice and speech data in PD, particularly utilizing DL models, highlight the role of AI-enhanced voice analysis as a valuable tool in clinical practice. This would help clinicians decide the management plans and prioritize the intervention procedures.

Most of the published studies targeted neurological disorder recognition in relation to healthy controls. There is a need for designing future studies discriminating different neurological disorders, even dysarthria subtypes, using AI models of voice analysis. Multimodality, including dysphagia markers along with voice features, possesses clinical interest. There are still several challenges that need to be addressed, including the development of user-friendly tools that do not require clinical settings and the enhancement of multilingual models to expand access to diverse populations.

Acknowledgments This chapter was inspired by a presentation originally delivered by Alberto Paderno at the Union of European Phoniatricians Committee on Biomarkers. The current text has been written by Neveen Hassan Nashaat, and any interpretations or elaborations are her own.

References

1. Steinmetz JD, Seeher KM, Schiess N, Nichols E, Cao B, Servili C, et al. Global, regional, and national burden of disorders affecting the nervous system, 1990–2021: a systematic analysis for the global burden of disease study 2021. Lancet Neurol. 2024;23(4):344–81. https://doi.org/10.1016/s1474-4422(24)00038-3.
2. Wang TV, Song PC. Neurological voice disorders: a review. Int J Head Neck Surg. 2022;13(1):32–40.
3. Hecker P, Steckhan N, Eyben F, Schuller BW, Arnrich B. Voice analysis for neurological disorder recognition – a systematic review and perspective on emerging trends. Front Digit Health. 2022;4:842301. https://doi.org/10.3389/fdgth.2022.842301.
4. Cummins N, Baird A, Schuller BW. Speech analysis for health: current state-of-the-art and the increasing impact of deep learning. Methods. 2018;1(151):41–54. https://doi.org/10.1016/j.ymeth.2018.07.007.
5. Toth L, Hoffmann I, Gosztolya G, Vincze V, Szatloczki G, Banreti Z, Pakaski M, Kalman J. A speech recognition-based solution for the automatic detection of mild cognitive impairment from spontaneous speech. Curr Alzheimer Res. 2018;15(2):130–8. https://doi.org/10.2174/1567205014666171121114930.
6. Aghanavesi S, Nyholm D, Senek M, Bergquist F, Memedi M. A smartphone-based system to quantify dexterity in Parkinson's disease patients. Inform Med Unlocked. 2017;9:11–7. https://doi.org/10.1016/j.imu.2017.05.005.

7. Alshammri R, Alharbi G, Alharbi E, Almubark I. Machine learning approaches to identify Parkinson's disease using voice signal features. Front Artif Intell. 2023;28(6):1084001. https://doi.org/10.3389/frai.2023.1084001.
8. Ahmed R, Hussein M, Keshk A. Comparative study of machine learning and deep learning algorithms for speech emotion recognition. Int J Comput Info. 2023;10(3) Proceedings of 2nd Int Conf on Comput & Info (ICCI), 83A
9. Karaman O, Çakın H, Alhudhaif A, Polat K. Robust automated Parkinson disease detection based on voice signals with transfer learning. Expert Syst Appl. 2021;178:115013. https://doi.org/10.1016/j.eswa.2021.115013.
10. de Jong NH, Pacilly J, Heeren W. PRAAT scripts to measure speed fluency and breakdown fluency in speech automatically. Assess Educ Princ Policy Pract. 2021;28(4):456–76. https://doi.org/10.1080/0969594X.2021.1951162.
11. Gnerre M, Malaspina E, Di Tella S, Anzuino I, Baglio F, Silveri MC, et al. Vocal emotional expression in Parkinson's disease: roles of sex and emotions. Societies. 2023;13(7):157. https://doi.org/10.3390/soc13070157.
12. Amiriparian S, Hübner T, Karas V, Gerczuk M, Ottl S, Schuller BW. DeepSpectrumLite: a Power-efficient transfer learning framework for embedded speech and audio processing from decentralized data. Front Artif Intell. 2022;5:856232. https://doi.org/10.3389/frai.2022.856232.
13. Berisha V, Liss JM. Responsible development of clinical speech AI: bridging the gap between clinical research and technology. NPJ Digit Med. 2024;7(1):208. https://doi.org/10.1038/s41746-024-01199-1.
14. Ding K, Chetty M, Hoshyar AN, Bhattacharya T, Klein B. Speech-based detection of Alzheimer's disease: a survey of AI techniques, datasets, and challenges. Artif Intell Rev. 2024;57:325–52. https://doi.org/10.1007/s10462-024-10961-6.
15. Freitag M, Amiriparian S, Pugachevskiy S, Cummins N, Schuller B. auDeep: unsupervised learning of representations from audio with deep recurrent neural networks. J Mach Learn Res. 2018;18:1–5. https://doi.org/10.48550/arXiv.1712.04382.
16. Haulcy R, Glass J. Classifying Alzheimer's disease using audio and text-based representations of speech. Front Psychol. 2021;11:624137. https://doi.org/10.3389/fpsyg.2020.624137.
17. Fristed E, Skirrow C, Meszaros M, Lenain R, Meepegama U, Cappa S, Aarsland D, Weston J. A remote speech-based AI system to screen for early Alzheimer's disease via smartphones. Alzheimers Dement (Amst). 2022;14:e12366. https://doi.org/10.1002/dad2.12366.
18. Agbavor F, Liang H. Predicting dementia from spontaneous speech using large language models. PLOS Digit Health. 2022;1:e0000168. https://doi.org/10.1371/journal.pdig.0000168.
19. Simmatis LER, Robin J, Spilka MJ, Yunusova Y. Detecting bulbar amyotrophic lateral sclerosis (ALS) using automatic acoustic analysis. Biomed Eng Online. 2024;23:15. https://doi.org/10.1186/s12938-023-01174-z.
20. Dubbioso R, Spisto M, Verde L, Iuzzolino VV, Senerchia G, Salvatore E, De Pietro G, De Falco I, Sannino G. Voice signals database of ALS patients with different dysarthria severity and healthy controls. Sci Data. 2024;11:800. https://doi.org/10.1038/s41597-024-03597-2.
21. Rong P, Yunusova Y, Wang J, Zinman L, Pattee GL, Berry JD, Perry B, Green JR. Predicting speech intelligibility decline in amyotrophic lateral sclerosis based on the deterioration of individual speech subsystems. PLoS One. 2016;11:e0154971. https://doi.org/10.1371/journal.pone.0154971.
22. Svoboda E, Bořil T, Rusz J, Tykalová T, Horáková D, Guttmann CRG, Blagoev KB, Hatabu H, Valtchinov VI. Assessing clinical utility of machine learning and artificial intelligence approaches to analyze speech recordings in multiple sclerosis: a pilot study. Comput Biol Med. 2022;148:105853. https://doi.org/10.1016/j.compbiomed.2022.105853.
23. Gosztolya G, Egas-López JV. Speech-based screening of multiple sclerosis by features derived from self-supervised models. In: International Conference on Electrical Computer and Energy Technologies (ICECET), Cape Town, South Africa, vol. 2023; 2023. p. 1–5. https://doi.org/10.1109/icecet58911.2023.10389218.
24. Sonkaya ZZ, Öztürk B, Sonkaya R, Taskiran E, Karadas Ö. Correction: Sonkaya et al. Using objective speech analysis techniques for the clinical diagnosis and assessment of speech dis-

orders in patients with multiple sclerosis. Brain Sci. 2024;14:384. Brain Sci 2024;14:1019. https://doi.org/10.3390/brainsci14101019.
25. Shimoda A, Li Y, Hayashi H, Kondo N. Dementia risks identified by vocal features via telephone conversations: a novel machine learning prediction model. PLoS One. 2021;16:e0253988. https://doi.org/10.1371/journal.pone.0253988.
26. Higuchi M, Nakamura M, Omiya Y, Tokuno S. Discrimination of mild cognitive impairment based on involuntary changes caused in voice elements. Front Neurol. 2023;14:1197840. https://doi.org/10.3389/fneur.2023.1197840.
27. Kashyap B, Pathirana PN, Horne M, Power L, Szmulewicz DJ. Machine learning-based scoring system to predict the risk and severity of ataxic speech using different speech tasks. IEEE Trans Neural Syst Rehabil Eng. 2023;31:4839–50. https://doi.org/10.1109/TNSRE.2023.3334718.
28. Isaev DY, Vlasova RM, Di Martino JM, Stephen CD, Schmahmann JD, Sapiro G, Gupta AS. Uncertainty of vowel predictions as a digital biomarker for ataxic dysarthria. Cerebellum. 2024;23:459–70. https://doi.org/10.1007/s12311-023-01539-z.
29. Song J, Lee JH, Choi J, Suh MK, Chung MJ, Kim YH, Park J, Choo SH, Son JH, Lee DY, Ahn JH, Youn J, Kim KS, Cho JW. Detection and differentiation of ataxic and hypokinetic dysarthria in cerebellar ataxia and parkinsonian disorders via wave splitting and integrating neural networks. PLoS One. 2022;17:e0268337. https://doi.org/10.1371/journal.pone.0268337.
30. Zhang Z, Yang LZ, Wang X, Li H. Automated detection of Wilson's disease based on improved Mel-frequency cepstral coefficients with signal decomposition. Proc Interspeech. 2022:2143–7. https://doi.org/10.21437/interspeech.2022-859.
31. Zhang Z, Yang LZ, Wang X, Wang H, Wong STC, Li H. Detecting Wilson's disease from unstructured connected speech: an embedding-based approach augmented by attention and bi-directional dependency. Speech Comm. 2024;156:103011. https://doi.org/10.1016/j.specom.2023.103011.
32. Rao Mv A, Yamini BK, Ketan J, Preetie Shetty A, Pal PK, Shivashankar N, Ghosh PK. Automatic classification of healthy subjects and patients with essential vocal tremor using probabilistic source-filter model based noise robust pitch estimation. J Voice. 2023;37:314–21. https://doi.org/10.1016/j.jvoice.2021.01.009.
33. Suppa A, Asci F, Saggio G, Di Leo P, Zarezadeh Z, Ferrazzano G, Ruoppolo G, Berardelli A, Costantini G. Voice analysis with machine learning: one step closer to an objective diagnosis of essential tremor. Mov Disord. 2021;36:1401–10. https://doi.org/10.1002/mds.28508.
34. Kouba T, Frank W, Tykalova T, Mühlbäck A, Klempíř J, Lindenberg KS, Landwehrmeyer GB, Rusz J. Speech biomarkers in Huntington's disease: a cross-sectional study in pre-symptomatic, prodromal and early manifest stages. Eur J Neurol. 2023;30:1262–71. https://doi.org/10.1111/ene.15726.
35. Nunes AS, Pawlik M, Mishra RK, Waddell E, Coffey M, Tarolli CG, Schneider RB, Dorsey ER, Vaziri A, Adams JL. Digital assessment of speech in Huntington disease. Front Neurol. 2024;15:1310548. https://doi.org/10.3389/fneur.2024.1310548.
36. Parekh N, Bhagat A, Raj B, Chhabra RS, Buttar HS, Kaur G, et al. Artificial intelligence in diagnosis and management of Huntington's disease. Beni-Suef Univ J Basic Appl Sci. 2023;12:87. https://doi.org/10.1186/s43088-023-00427-z.
37. Ramesh S, Arachchige ASPM. Depletion of dopamine in Parkinson's disease and relevant therapeutic options: a review of the literature. AIMS Neurosci. 2023;10:200–31. https://doi.org/10.3934/Neuroscience.2023017.
38. Rusz J, Cmejla R, Tykalova T, Ruzickova H, Klempir J, Majerova V, Picmausova J, Roth J, Ruzicka E. Imprecise vowel articulation as a potential early marker of Parkinson's disease: effect of speaking task. J Acoust Soc Am. 2013;134:2171–81. https://doi.org/10.1121/1.4816541.
39. Huang X, Wang F, Gao Y, Liao Y, Zhang W, Zhang L, Xu Z. Depression recognition using voice-based pre-training model. Sci Rep. 2024;14:12734. https://doi.org/10.1038/s41598-024-63556-0.
40. Shin D, Cho WI, Park CHK, Rhee SJ, Kim MJ, Lee H, Kim NS, Ahn YM. Detection of minor and major depression through voice as a biomarker using machine learning. J Clin Med. 2021;10:3046. https://doi.org/10.3390/jcm10143046.

41. Tyagi S, Szénási S. Semantic speech analysis using machine learning and deep learning techniques: a comprehensive review. Multimed Tools Appl. 2024;83:73427–56. https://doi.org/10.1007/s11042-023-17769-6.
42. Gauder L, Riera P, Slachevsky A, Forno G, Garcia AM, Ferrer L. The unreliability of acoustic systems in Alzheimer's speech datasets with heterogeneous recording conditions. ArXiv. 2024:abs/2409.12170. https://doi.org/10.48550/arXiv.2409.12170.
43. Paaß G, Giesselbach S. Foundation models for speech, images, videos, and control. In: Foundation models for natural language processing. Artificial intelligence: foundations, theory, and algorithms. Cham: Springer; 2023. p. 313–82. https://doi.org/10.1007/978-3-031-23190-2_7.
44. Zaman K, Sah M, Direkoglu C, Unoki M. A survey of audio classification using deep learning. IEEE Access. 2023;11:106620–49. https://doi.org/10.1109/access.2023.3318015.
45. Bertini F, Allevi D, Lutero G, Calza L, Montesi D. A cross-language dementia classifier: a preliminary study. In: 2022 IEEE int conf metrol ext real, AI& neural eng. (MetroXRAINE), vol. 2022. IEEE. p. 438–43. https://doi.org/10.1109/metroxraine54828.2022.9967558.
46. Costantini G, Cesarini V, Di Leo P, Amato F, Suppa A, Asci F, Pisani A, Calculli A, Saggio G. Artificial intelligence-based voice assessment of patients with Parkinson's disease off and on treatment: machine vs. deep-learning comparison. Sensors. 2023;23:2293. https://doi.org/10.3390/s23042293.
47. Suppa A, Costantini G, Gomez-Vilda P, Saggio G. Editorial: voice analysis in healthy subjects and patients with neurologic disorders. Front Neurol. 2023;14:1288370. https://doi.org/10.3389/fneur.2023.1288370.

Open Access This chapter is licensed under the terms of the Creative Commons Attribution-NonCommercial-NoDerivatives 4.0 International License (http://creativecommons.org/licenses/by-nc-nd/4.0/), which permits any noncommercial use, sharing, distribution and reproduction in any medium or format, as long as you give appropriate credit to the original author(s) and the source, provide a link to the Creative Commons license and indicate if you modified the licensed material. You do not have permission under this license to share adapted material derived from this chapter or parts of it.

The images or other third party material in this chapter are included in the chapter's Creative Commons license, unless indicated otherwise in a credit line to the material. If material is not included in the chapter's Creative Commons license and your intended use is not permitted by statutory regulation or exceeds the permitted use, you will need to obtain permission directly from the copyright holder.

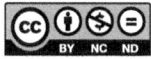

Modeling a Preclinical Screening Tool Based on Voice-Related Biomarkers: The Case of Parkinson's Disease

Ramón Hernández-Villoria

4.1 Introduction

4.1.1 What Would Be a Screening Tool Based on Voice-Related Biomarkers?

According to the biomarkers' definition, they must indicate a process's normal or pathological state. For at least a decade, there has been interest in finding early indicators of illness—or health recovery—in the voice. Voice is the sound resulting from the complex interaction of several processes. Intuitively, we all know that in different diseases, the characteristics of the human voice are perceptually altered. Diseases of the vocal folds or the laryngeal vestibule cause voice alteration, but pulmonary, cardiovascular, endocrine, psychiatric, and neurological pathological processes can also generate changes in vocal production that can eventually be identified even very early in the onset of the disease or a change of stage. It is even possible to do it outside of an office, with telemedicine or Mobile Health (mHealth) tools, perceptually and acoustically analyzing the voice signal [1].

Inclusion Within the Concept of Biomarkers Traditionally, biomarkers arise from the chemical analysis and identification of substances or molecules in tissues and fluids by different means. Kraus [2] points out that developing a biomarker is a multi-step and iterative process, from its discovery as a candidate to its qualification and clinical use.

According to Fagherazzi et al. [3], a vocal biomarker is "a signature, a feature, or a combination of features from the **audio signal**." It is associated with a clinical

---

R. Hernández-Villoria (✉)
Centro Clínico de Audición y Lenguaje Cealca, Caracas, Venezuela

Hospital de Clínicas Caracas, Caracas, Venezuela

© The Author(s) 2026
M. Pedersen et al. (eds.), *Voice-related Biomarkers*,
https://doi.org/10.1007/978-3-032-03134-1_4

expression, so it can be used to diagnose, monitor the evolution, or classify a disease's stage or degree of severity. They even propose that it could be used for drug development, just like any other type of biomarker. Vocal biomarkers deviate from the traditional taxonomy of biomarkers since neither tissue nor fluid is analyzed. Vocal biomarkers fall into the category of digital biomarkers since the computer analysis of a physical element (sound) provides numerical indicators that represent physical behaviors from which a particular state is deduced.

Increasing Use of Voice-Related Biomarkers The first attempts to obtain reliable indicators of psychiatric disorders based on speech or voice samples date back to the 1970s [4]. However, even with the improvements in computerized acoustic voice analysis in the 1990s, there was no great success in specifying univocal correlations between acoustic parameters and changes in the vocal fold tissue itself, much less in multifactorial situations such as psychiatric ones [5].

Later, more significant consideration was given to the acoustic features of the voice as markers of depression and anxiety [6]. Neurology is also interested in this type of indicator for the early detection of Huntington's [7], Parkinson's [8], and Alzheimer's [9]. Artificial intelligence has improved the use of voice-related biomarkers. The boom in telemedicine during the COVID-19 pandemic led to interest in having tools available to identify early changes associated with SARS-CoV-2 infection through voice over the telephone [10].

A section has been opened on the taxonomy of biomarkers since they will no longer be based exclusively on biochemistry. Voice-related biomarkers would be very inexpensive, noninvasive, and widely available.

4.1.2 The Central Problem of Voice as a Biomarker

Some authors have pointed out the challenge of identifying voice-related biomarker candidates. The correlation of acoustic parameters does not accurately inform which specific alteration of the vocal folds may be occurring. On the other hand, as in the process of standardizing and accepting the reliability of a biochemical biomarker, the voice-related biomarker must undergo a long process of testing, iteration, and verification.

It is essential to consider the voice as a multidimensional phenomenon, not only evaluable by its acoustic aspect. The European Laryngological Society and the Union of European Phoniatricians have highlighted the multidimensional concept in consensus [11]. The voice's multidimensionality means that the relationship or combination between parameters of the different dimensions must be taken into account to arrive at a correct evaluation of the voice with the highest sensitivity and specificity.

4.1.3 Screening Tools

According to the World Health Organization [12], health screening tools must have the following characteristics: they must be low cost, easy to implement, safe, and widely available. In addition, they must be able to identify diseases with significant prevalence in the asymptomatic period when applying a treatment that would reduce or prevent future morbidity and mortality. For this, an effective treatment must be identified. The screening tool must have high statistical sensitivity and specificity.

As noted, using the values of physical parameters in the voice or their combinations as biomarkers has excellent advantages related to the meager cost and ease of obtaining the sample, signal processing and analysis using software, ease of storage and distribution, and reproducibility in different analysis environments. The increasing and more widespread quality of cell phone devices in the general public, with sufficiently qualified microphones and processors, generates the suitability of using the voice as a screening tool worldwide. The challenge is to systematize identifying the most minor and most subtle changes in physical values and what combinations of these changes occur in different diseases and health conditions and their alteration, including in prodromal stages, in which screening would increase its importance to guarantee early intervention.

4.1.4 Parkinson's Disease and Voice-Related Screening as an Example

It is well established that Parkinson's Disease (PD), a neurodegenerative disease, causes audibly perceptible voice changes once it has already set in. These changes have been described as hypophonia, monotony, and tremor [13].

The proposal to identify PD early follows the idea that this could allow very early intervention and slow down the worsening of the disease. Voice-related tools help identify successive disease stages or the success of pharmacological interventions.

The pathophysiological basis of using the voice as an indicator of early PD-related changes comes from the structure of the vocal folds, which are the main biological elements for voice production. The intrinsic muscles are susceptible to small perturbations of contraction, both isotonic and isometric. See Fig. 4.1.

PD is characterized by bradykinesia (slowness in movement execution), akinesia (difficulty initiating movement, observed as rigidity), and hypometria (failure to develop the amplitude of movement). These features, applied to the intrinsic musculature of the vocal folds, may explain the most common findings (see Table 4.1). In Parkinsonism, hypo-adduction of the vocal folds is the most frequent finding [13].

Other vocal symptoms of established PD are hypophonia (a soft, exhaled voice of low intensity) and monotony (difficulty varying the pitch or frequency of vibration of the vocal folds when speaking). Since hypophonia corresponds to low glottal pressure, it can be attributed to the disease's effects on the respiratory musculature, while monotony is due to akinesia at a more advanced stage.

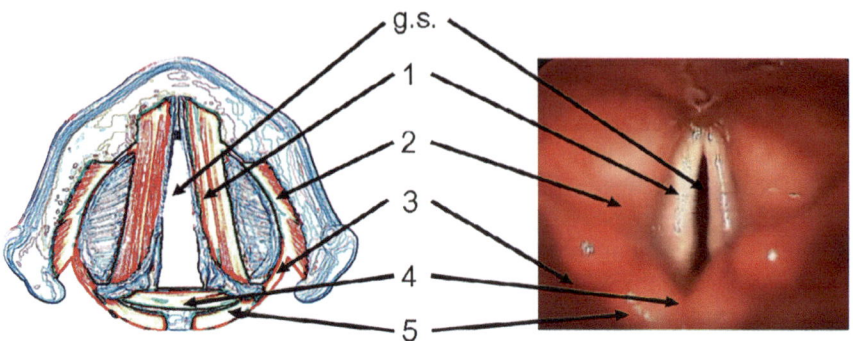

Fig. 4.1 Schematic view of the intrinsic laryngeal musculature and actual endoscopic view of the endolarynx. This figure shows glottal space (g.s.); muscles: *1.* thyroarytenoid. *2.* cricothyroid. *3.* lateral cricoarytenoid. *4.* interarytenoid. *5.* posterior cricoarytenoid. On the right is an actual picture, obtained from laryngeal endoscopy, in which the plane of the glottis and vocal cords is observed from above. On the left, a schematic drawing of the same plane allows us to observe the position of the intrinsic muscles and cartilaginous skeleton of the larynx

Resting tremor, with a frequency of 4 to 7 Hz, is a late-stage feature. Vocal tremor, according to Tykalová et al. [14], is low in prevalence, independent of the PD variant, and isolated from limb tremor. The trembling effect on the voice would not be due to tremors in the moving vocal folds, but rather due to the resting tremor of other muscles in the laryngopharyngeal tract that modify the harmonic frequencies of the voice.

Impairment of intrinsic and extrinsic laryngeal muscle function and respiratory musculature will result in measurable physical changes in the acoustics of the projected vocal sound. Thus, acoustic voice analysis and glottal inverse filtering (GIF) provide information about subtle changes in these muscular dynamics.

4.2 Perspectives

4.2.1 Contextualizing Voice Parameters: The Case of Parkinson's Disease

Diagnosis and Stages of PD Despite the intensive search for biomarkers, PD continues to be diagnosed clinically. It is based on the conjunction of two or more symptoms/signs: bradykinesia, akinesia (muscle rigidity), resting tremor, and postural instability. Concordance with postmortem histopathological diagnosis varies between 75% and 99% [15].

According to the consensus of the Movement Disorders Society (MDS), PD develops in stages: (i) preclinical stage, (ii) prodromal stage, and (iii) clinical disease. In the preclinical stage, degenerative changes in the substantia nigra have begun, but no symptoms or signs are evident. The prodromal stage includes the

Table 4.1 Basal motor and derived vocal symptoms, biomechanics involved, and probable acoustic changes in Parkinson's disease

Basal motor symptom	Derived vocal symptom	Biomechanics involved	Probable acoustic changes
Bradykinesia	Breathy sound	Vocal fold hypoadduction	HNR reduction
			GNE increasing
	Hypophonia (low intensity)	Low subglottic pressure	Mean SPL reduction
			NNE increasing
			HNR reduction
	Monoloudness (no variation in loudness when talking)	Reduction in the respiratory muscles' motion range	VRP reduction
			shimmer increasing
	Mono pitch (no variation in pitch when talking)	Difficulty in modifying the length and mass of the vocal folds	F0 no change
			Jitter increasing
			VRP reduction
Akinesia	Glottal stop at onset	Difficulty initiating adduction	Reduced pitch variation
			VRP reduced
			GNE increase
Resting tremor	Quavering voice	Tremor in the throat muscles	F0 fluctuation
			MDFT increase
			MDAT increase

Lists the three main motor symptoms of Parkinson's disease and the corresponding consequences, such as vocal symptoms, laryngeal biomechanics, and acoustic changes in the voice of each of them
HNR harmonic-to-noise ratio, *GNE* glottal noise energy, *VRP* voice range profile, *SPL* sound pressure level, *NNE* noise normalized energy, *F0* fundamental frequency, *MDFT* modulation depth of frequency tremor, *MDAT* modulation depth of amplitude tremor

appearance of symptoms and signs of neurodegeneration at both the non-motor and motor levels. In the clinical stage, bradykinesia becomes evident and is accompanied by either rigidity or tremor, as already described.

Figure 4.2 shows a gradual transition from the preclinical to the prodromal stage. People with genetics for PD and exposure to risk factors will develop the prodromal stage generally in their 40s or 50s. They may develop clinical symptoms ten to fifteen years later when the diagnosis is verifiable. See the list of non-motor and motor symptoms in Table 4.2.

Voice Studies in the Different Stages of PD Voice characteristics in the different clinical stages and during treatment with L-DOPA [16, 17] have been well studied and described. Holmes et al. mention that the voice is limited to varying the pitch and the sonority. Characteristically, the voice has "breathiness, harshness, and

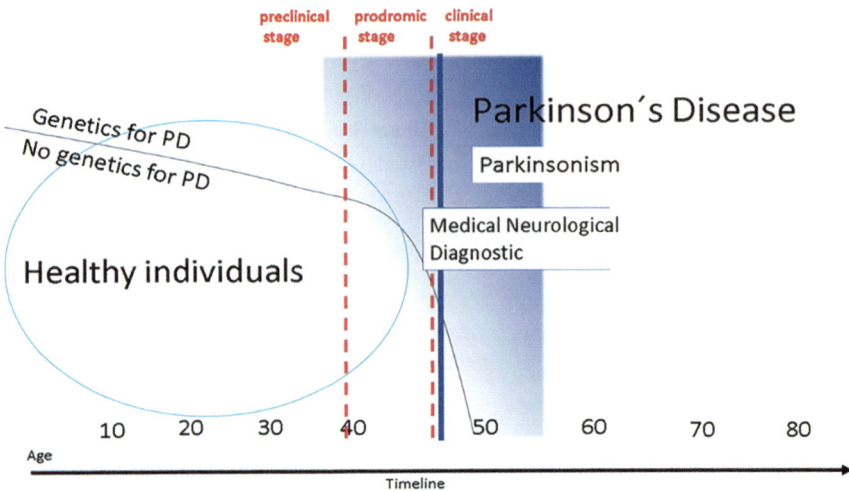

Fig. 4.2 Parkinson's disease timeline (age), course, and stages. This figure shows the timeline in decades of life (age) of the most relevant moments in the natural history of Parkinson's disease. The vertically dotted red lines delimit the approximate times between the disease's preclinical, prodromal, and clinical stages. The blue shade tells us how flowery the symptoms are expressed. Based on the clinic, the neurological medical diagnosis is usually made when the symptoms are very evident (between the end of the prodromal stage and the beginning of the clinical stage, demarcated by the solid vertical blue line). On the left, healthy individuals or those with the disease without PD genetics are less likely to show symptoms than those with PD genetics

Table 4.2 Parkinson's disease. Prodromal symptoms and signs

No motor symptoms	Motor symptoms (very subtle changes)
Rapid eye movement sleep disorders	Voice production
Anosmia	Finger skills
Constipation	Altered arm movement
Depression	Altered gait (steps)

Lists the most common non-motor and motor symptoms in the prodromal stage of Parkinson's disease

reduced loudness." Furthermore, the advanced stage is characterized by high modal pitch levels in males. According to these authors, most of the characteristics do not increase the deterioration with the worsening of the disease, but "breathiness, monopitch and monoloudness, and low loudness" do. Also, the phonatory frequency range reduction worsens in the later stages of PD. On the other hand, tremor is the only characteristic associated with the advanced stage of PD.

Vocal symptoms appear very early in the course of the disease [18]. It was found that around 80% of people with PD in the early clinical stage, prior to any pharmacological or speech therapy intervention, present vocal and acoustic alterations, even if they do not have obvious perceptual manifestations in the voice and can be separated from healthy controls when studying the acoustic parameters.

Postuma [8] concludes, after reviewing research on voice acoustics in PD, that "the voice changes are among the most robust motor abnormalities" and that voice changes could separate the group with PD in the prodromal stage from the group of healthy controls. Studies by Rusz et al. [18, 19] finds it possible to differentiate a group of people with idiopathic rapid eye movement sleep behavior disorder (RBD) from controls without RBD. According to the study, the acoustic parameters linked to airflow insufficiency, irregular pitch fluctuations, signal perturbations, and aperiodicity are the most marked.

4.2.2 Multidimensional Voice Model and Acoustic Measurement

The voice is a biological sound with multiple dimensions. The European Laryngology Society-Union of European Phoniatricians (ELS-UEP) 2023 consensus [11] suggests a seven-dimensional model for voice assessment. A summary of these dimensions is in Table 4.3.

Multidimensional Voice Model in PD A family history of PD and PD risk factors should be collected in the baseline anamnesis to build the screening model for the disease in its preclinical or prodromal stage.

Videolaryngostroboscopy. Some articles describe the following changes observed in PD: incomplete or asymmetric glottic closure, hypoadduction, and bowing of the vocal folds [20]. The more advanced the disease, the more noticeable these changes become. However, increased phase asymmetry is the best-validated videostroboscopic marker [21]. More subtle findings are asymmetrical in the movement of the arytenoid cartilages and increased glottal opening time.

Table 4.3 Minimum Voice Quality Assessment based upon ESL-UEP Consensus

Dimension	Minimum parameters in the preclinical evaluation of PD
Baseline anamnesis	Allergy, medical and surgical history, medication, addiction, singing practice, job, and posture
Videolaryngostroboscopy	Phase asymmetry
Patient-reported voice quality assessment	Voice handicap index (VHI-30, VHI-10)
Perception	GRBAS-visual analogue scale
Aerodynamics	Maximum phonation time (MPT)
Acoustics	Mean F0, jitter, shimmer, HNR
Clinical instruments associated with voice comorbidities	Reflux Symptom Score, Reflux Sign Assessment, Eating Assessment Tool-10, Dysphagia Handicap Index

The correspondence between the dimensions of the 7D model of voice quality evaluation according to the ELS-UEP and the minimum parameters to be evaluated in each dimension
F0 fundamental frequency, *HNR* harmonics to noise ratio

Self-assessment. Voice Handicap Index-30 (VHI-30) is preferable over the simplified VHI-10 since, in PD, the emotional and social components of the voice over time may be better represented. Self-assessment with a Visual Analogue Scale (VAS) at baseline is also helpful.

Aerodynamics. The maximum phonation time (MPT) is a parameter consistently altered in all stages of PD, but other parameters, such as the direct measurement of mean sound pressure in decibels of sound pressure level and the indirect measurement of mean phonatory resistance, have shown their utility in the study of PD. A separate chapter of aerodynamics is the glottal inverse filter (GIF) analysis, discussed in another chapter of this volume. In addition, the GIF allows for more extensive use by expanding it with the application of AI.

Perceptual assessment. The GRBAS scale (grade, roughness, breathiness, asthenia, strain), the most widespread and used worldwide, is not in question for documenting the perceptual variable of vocal quality. It is advisable to use the VAS version of the scale.

Comorbidities. Using clinical questionnaires for comorbidity is a very interesting point in PD. They provide the possibility to exclude confusing causes of subtle changes in acoustic parameters, such as gastroesophageal-laryngeal reflux, which is not directly related to PD. In addition, they would contribute to delving into another prodromal symptom: dysphagia, since subtle dysphagic symptoms could be considered as early as vocal changes [22].

Acoustic measurements of the voice. There are many PD and acoustic voice analysis studies, which we will not list here. Of all the parameters, the most studied have been the fundamental frequency (F0) and its standard deviation (F0 SD), jitter %, intensity, shimmer, and harmonic-to-noise ratio (HNR) or the inverse noise to the harmonic ratio (NHR). To a lesser extent, studies have been published with the parameters Long Time Average Spectrum (LTAS), Signal to Noise Ratio (SNR), Cepstrum Peak Prominence (CPP), and Voice Range Profile (VRP). Other parameters that were studied and validated as indicators of changes associated with PD are glottal-to-noise excitation ratio (GNE), normalized pitch period entropy (norm PPE), detrended fluctuation analysis (DFA), and glottal closing quotient (ClQ)—which is an aerodynamic parameter measurable by acoustic means.

The short-term parameters measure sound perturbation cycle by cycle. In dysphonic periodic voice, the short-term perturbation parameters are more altered the more advanced the disease (i.e., inflammatory, degenerative, etc.), until the voice turns into an aperiodic one.

There is a continuum from normal voice to aperiodic voice through dysphonic periodic voice. In preclinical or prodromic PD, what we want to detect with screening is closer to normal than dysphonia; therefore, short-term parameters might not be altered yet.

In contrast, long-term (or overall) parameters would be more helpful in detecting subtle and incipient changes, as occurs in other voice screening situations, such as occupational voice screening. Long-term parameters measure the variations in a set of examined signals as a variable (e.g., periodic energy) within the set decays or increases.

Some of the long-term parameters that have been considered in different studies have been the Long-Time Average Spectrum (LTAS), cepstral peak prominence (CPP), and all its related variant parameters, including mel frequency cepstral coefficients (MFCC).

There are also slightly more complex acoustic parameter values, such as Fractal Dimension (FD) and Normalized Mutual Information (NMI), that examine the sound of the voice, with which some studies of pathological voice in PD have been carried out [23].

4.2.3 Other PD Screening Tools Not Based on Voice But Linked to Bradykinesia

Tools Based on Facial Hypomimia Methods for identifying subtle bradykinetic motor changes based on hypomimia or decreased facial mimic have also been sought [24].

After evaluating different natural facial movements (not in specific tasks), they paid particular attention to the potential of blink measurement, such as a blink frequency over 30 s [25]. These last authors propose the integration, in a biometric tool, of blink measurement with voice measurements in a speech task.

Using the integrated blink/voice-speech tool in a group of early-stage PD cases compared to a group of healthy controls and combining it with a deep learning classifier has found a statistically significant value for its ability to differentiate between the two groups.

Tools Based on Acoustic Pharyngometry Bradykinesia compromises the mobility of the arytenoid cartilage in the early stages of PD. Mobility of the cartilages is a kinetic expression of the contractility of the posterior cricoarytenoid and lateral cricoarytenoid muscles, which abduct and adduct, respectively, the arytenoids and, therefore, the vocal folds, opening or closing the glottic space and increasing or decreasing the glottic area. These movements and changes are relevant not only for voice production but also for swallowing.

Videolaryngostroboscopy can measure these changes in the glottis and arytenoids, but it is an invasive examination. Computed tomography (CT) has been used to measure interarytenoid distance, even in patients with PD, without invading the patient [26], but it is an expensive study with ionizing radiation.

A less invasive alternative is acoustic pharyngometry, a study that measures the reflection of sound waves in the oropharyngeal tract to measure its volume. It has been successfully used to find differences in the size of the glottal area in patients with PD compared to healthy controls [27]. These authors also consider combining acoustic pharyngometry with acoustic voice parameters as a PD screening tool.

4.3 Discussion

Developing a PD screening tool based on voice-related biomarkers must consider several aspects. First, it must detect minimal and subtle changes that clearly point to PD's earliest motor feature, bradykinesia. Bradykinesia, which affects the intrinsic laryngeal muscles that control the precision of vocal fold movement and, therefore, the final result of the voice, can be deduced precisely from the cycle-by-cycle perturbation and also from the changes in sonority over a long period, even before these changes are perceptible or measurable in connected speech.

Various acoustic parameters help differentiate statistically significant groups of PD in the early stages from groups of healthy controls. However, in the early stage, the clinical diagnosis is already made. There is more interest in identifying the PD group in the prodromal stage when non-motor symptoms can generate diagnostic confusion. Identification is even more interesting when the disease is in the preclinical stage and there are no recognizable motor or non-motor symptoms.

Any screening tool should only be considered part of a broader concept: the screening program. The program should describe the population at risk for the disease. It is known that only a small percentage of PD has a familial character, but some genetic traits are relevant to risk factors. The phenotypic expressions of PD can be broader than those traditionally recognized as characteristics of the disease, and this causes difficulties in identifying which group is at risk. Conducting population genetic studies, even to identify a few genes, is very expensive.

Some authors performed risk factor studies to identify increasingly large sets of factors. Ascherio and Schwarzschild [28] report that the main ones are exposure to pesticides, consumption of dairy products, history of melanoma, and history of head trauma. In a rigorous study, Shi et al. [29] identified 27 risk factors by analyzing phenotypes and genotypes of more than five hundred thousand subjects from the UK Biobank. These findings help to better define the landscape for designing studies with voice-related biomarkers that detect possible subjects developing PD in the preclinical stage.

Another element to consider is that the voice is not only its acoustic dimension, which is already complex and difficult to summarize in a single parameter. The voice must also be measured in its perceptual and aerodynamic dimensions, in addition to collecting an anamnesis that examines the intervening factors that affect the voice and information on comorbidities. These dimensions are examined through the analysis of the voice signal and remote answering of questionnaires.

The relationship between the values of parameters extracted from the vocal sound and the biomechanics of the larynx deserves special mention. Biomechanics is studied visually using video stroboscopy, an invasive and medium-cost medical procedure, which is why it would be excluded from the first screening phase. Other biomechanical indicators could represent less invasive alternatives, such as the aforementioned acoustic pharyngometry, which would require additional equipment and not measure the phase asymmetry of the mucosal wave but rather another indicator, the glottal area. Instead, mucosal wave phase asymmetry can be measured indirectly by acoustic techniques based on a glottal inverse filter (GIF) that only needs to capture the speech signal.

4.4 Conclusions

The modeling of a preclinical identification tool centered on using a voice-related biomarker must start from validation in a risk group for PD versus a control group without these risk factors. The biomarker must consider a multidimensional and multiparametric framework within each dimension, as demonstrated by the findings of many strictly acoustic voice studies in early PD. There are parameters already studied and validated to identify PD; it is only necessary to integrate them into a single instrument and verify them in the prodromal and preclinical stages. A first phase of a screening program is even feasible by mHealth, conveniently capturing the voice signal necessary for analysis in the perceptual, acoustic, and aerodynamic dimensions, and indirectly an equivalent of the laryngostroboscopic dimension, which is actually a biomechanical dimension. The dimensions related to anamnesis, comorbidity, and voice handicap index can also be integrated into an mHealth solution, making the proper development of a tool based on a voice-related biomarker feasible. Interestingly, when studying other possible biomarkers, the combination with voice-related biomarkers is always suggested for the early detection of PD.

References

1. Sara JDS, Orbelo D, Maor E, Lerman LO, Lerman A. Guess what we can hear – voice biomarkers for the novel remote detection of disease. Mayo Clin Proc. 2023;98:1353–75. https://doi.org/10.1016/j.mayocp.2023.03.007.
2. Kraus VB. Biomarkers as drug development tools: discovery, validation, qualification and use. Nat Rev Rheumatol. 2018;14:354–62. https://doi.org/10.1038/s41584-018-0005-9.
3. Fagherazzi G, Fischer A, Ismael M, Despotovic V. Voice for health: the use of vocal biomarkers from research to clinical practice. Digit Biomark. 2021;5:78–88. https://doi.org/10.1159/000515346.
4. Darby JK, Hollien H. Vocal and speech patterns of depressive patients. Folia Phoniatr (Basel). 1977;29:279–91. https://doi.org/10.1159/000264098.
5. Mendoza E, Carballo G. Acoustic analysis of induced vocal stress by means of cognitive workload tasks. J Voice. 1998;12:263–73. https://doi.org/10.1016/s0892-1997(98)80017-9.
6. Cannizzaro M, Harel B, Reilly N, Chappell P, Snyder PJ. Voice acoustical measurement of the severity of major depression. Brain Cogn. 2004;56:30–5. https://doi.org/10.1016/j.bandc.2004.05.003.
7. Rusz J, Saft C, Schlegel U, Hoffman R, Skodda S. Phonatory dysfunction as a preclinical symptom of Huntington disease. PLoS One. 2014;9:e113412. https://doi.org/10.1371/journal.pone.0113412.
8. Postuma RB. Voice changes in prodromal Parkinson's disease: is a new biomarker within earshot? Sleep Med. 2016;19:148–9. https://doi.org/10.1016/j.sleep.2015.08.019.
9. Martínez-Sánchez F, Meilán JJG, Carro J, Ivanova O. A prototype for the voice analysis diagnosis of Alzheimer's disease. J Alzheimers Dis. 2018;64(2):473–81. https://doi.org/10.3233/JAD-180037.

10. Maor E, Tsur N, Barkai G, Meister I, Makmel S, Friedman E, Aronovich D, Mevorach D, Lerman A, Zimlichman E, Bachar G. Noninvasive vocal biomarker is associated with severe acute respiratory syndrome coronavirus 2 infection. Mayo Clin Proc Innov Qual Outcomes. 2021;5:654–62. https://doi.org/10.1016/j.mayocpiqo.2021.05.007.
11. Lechien JR, Geneid A, Bohlender JE, Cantarella G, Avellaneda JC, Desuter G, et al. Consensus for voice quality assessment in clinical practice: guidelines of the European Laryngological Society and Union of the European Phoniatricians. Eur Arch Otorhinolaryngol. 2023;280:5459–73. https://doi.org/10.1007/s00405-023-08211-6.
12. World Health Organization. Regional Office for Europe. Screening programmes: a short guide. Increase effectiveness, maximize benefits and minimize harm. Regional Office for Europe. World Health Organization; 2020. Available from: https://iris.who.int/handle/10665/330829
13. Rubin J, Shields K. Central neurogenic voice disorders. In: Am Zehnhoff-Dinnesen A, Wiskirska-Woźnica B, Neumann K, Nawka T, editors. Phoniatrics I: fundamentals, voice disorders, disorders of language and hearing development. 1st ed. Berlin: Springer; 2020. p. 271–80. (European Manual of Medicine).
14. Tykalová T, Rusz J, Švihlík J, Bancone S, Spezia A, Pellecchia MT. Speech disorder and vocal tremor in postural instability/gait difficulty and tremor dominant subtypes of Parkinson's disease. J Neural Transm (Vienna). 2020;127:1295–304. https://doi.org/10.1007/s00702-020-02229-4.
15. Postuma RB, Berg D. The new diagnostic criteria for Parkinson's disease. Int Rev Neurobiol. 2017;132:55–78. https://doi.org/10.1016/bs.irn.2017.01.008.
16. Holmes RJ, Oates JM, Phyland DJ, Hughes AJ. Voice characteristics in the progression of Parkinson's disease. Int J Lang Commun Disord. 2000;35:407–18. https://doi.org/10.1080/136828200410654.
17. Lechien JR, Blecic S, Huet K, Delvaux V, Piccaluga M, Roland V, Harmegnies B, Saussez S. Voice quality outcomes of idiopathic Parkinson's disease medical treatment: a systematic review. Clin Otolaryngol. 2018;43:882–903. https://doi.org/10.1111/coa.13082.
18. Rusz J, Cmejla R, Ruzickova H, Ruzicka E. Quantitative acoustic measurements for characterization of speech and voice disorders in early untreated Parkinson's disease. J Acoust Soc Am. 2011;129:350–67. https://doi.org/10.1121/1.3514381.
19. Rusz J, Hlavnička J, Tykalová T, Bušková J, Ulmanová O, Růžička E, Šonka K. Quantitative assessment of motor speech abnormalities in idiopathic rapid eye movement sleep behaviour disorder. Sleep Med. 2016;19:141–7. https://doi.org/10.1016/j.sleep.2015.07.030.
20. Yücetürk AV, Yilmaz H, Eğrilmez M, Karaca S. Voice analysis and videolaryngostroboscopy in patients with Parkinson's disease. Eur Arch Otorhinolaryngol. 2002;259:290–3. https://doi.org/10.1007/s00405-002-0462-1.
21. Ma A, Lau KK, Thyagarajan D. Voice changes in Parkinson's disease: what are they telling us? J Clin Neurosci. 2020;72:1–7. https://doi.org/10.1016/j.jocn.2019.12.029.
22. Wang P, Chen X, Chen M, Gao L, Xiong B, Ji C, et al. Dysphagia pattern in early to moderate Parkinson's disease caused by abnormal pharyngeal kinematic function. Dysphagia. 2024;39:905–15. https://doi.org/10.1007/s00455-024-10672-8.
23. Viswanathan R, Arjunan SP, Bingham A, Jelfs B, Kempster P, Raghav S, Kumar DK. Complexity measures of voice recordings as a discriminative tool for Parkinson's disease. Biosensors (Basel). 2019;10:1. https://doi.org/10.3390/bios10010001.
24. Maycas-Cepeda T, López-Ruiz P, Feliz-Feliz C, Gómez-Vicente L, García-Cobos R, Arroyo R, García-Ruiz PJ. Hypomimia in Parkinson's disease: what is it telling us? Front Neurol. 2021;11:603582. https://doi.org/10.3389/fneur.2020.603582.
25. Lim WS, Chiu SI, Wu MC, Tsai SF, Wang PH, Lin KP, et al. An integrated biometric voice and facial features for early detection of Parkinson's disease. NPJ Parkinsons Dis. 2022:8. https://doi.org/10.1038/s41531-022-00414-8.
26. Perju-Dumbrava L, Lau K, Phyland D, Papanikolaou V, Finlay P, Beare R, et al. Arytenoid cartilage movements are hypokinetic in Parkinson's disease: a quantitative dynamic computerised tomographic study. PLoS One. 2017;12:e0186611. https://doi.org/10.1371/journal.pone.0186611.

27. Curtis JA, Molfenter SM, Troche MS. Pharyngeal area changes in Parkinson's disease and its effect on swallowing safety, efficiency, and kinematics. Dysphagia. 2020;35(2):389–98. https://doi.org/10.1007/s00455-019-10052-7.
28. Ascherio A, Schwarzschild MA. The epidemiology of Parkinson's disease: risk factors and prevention. Lancet Neurol. 2016;15:1257–72. https://doi.org/10.1016/S1474-4422(16)30230-7.
29. Shi C, Ma D, Li M, Wang Z, Hao C, Liang Y, et al. Identifying potential causal effects of Parkinson's disease: a polygenic risk score-based phenome-wide association and Mendelian randomization study in UK Biobank. NPJ Parkinsons Dis. 2024:10. https://doi.org/10.1038/s41531-024-00780-5.

Open Access   This chapter is licensed under the terms of the Creative Commons Attribution-NonCommercial-NoDerivatives 4.0 International License (http://creativecommons.org/licenses/by-nc-nd/4.0/), which permits any noncommercial use, sharing, distribution and reproduction in any medium or format, as long as you give appropriate credit to the original author(s) and the source, provide a link to the Creative Commons license and indicate if you modified the licensed material. You do not have permission under this license to share adapted material derived from this chapter or parts of it.

The images or other third party material in this chapter are included in the chapter's Creative Commons license, unless indicated otherwise in a credit line to the material. If material is not included in the chapter's Creative Commons license and your intended use is not permitted by statutory regulation or exceeds the permitted use, you will need to obtain permission directly from the copyright holder.

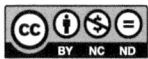

Glottal Inverse Filtering and Its Application in the Automatic Classification of Diseases from Speech

5

Paavo Alku, Ramón Hernández-Villoria, and Sneha Das

5.1 Introduction

Glottal inverse filtering (GIF) is a technique used to estimate the source of voiced speech, the glottal volume velocity, from the speech pressure signal recorded by a microphone (or from the oral flow recorded by a flow mask). Most GIF methods are based on the linear source–filter model of speech production (Fig. 5.1). According to this simplified model, speech is produced as a cascade of three processes (the glottal flow, vocal tract, and lip radiation effect). Using computational models for the filtering effects of the vocal tract and lip radiation, the effects of these two processes can be cancelled from the speech signal by filtering the recorded signal through the inverses of the vocal tract and lip radiation model (Fig. 5.2). In other words, GIF aims to estimate the input of the voice production system, that is, the glottal excitation, when the output, that is, the speech signal, is known. Computational models for the vocal tract and lip radiation are typically implemented as digital

---

P. Alku
Department of Information and Communications Engineering, Aalto University, Espoo, Finland
e-mail: paavo.alku@aalto.fi

R. Hernández-Villoria (✉)
Centro Clínico de Audición y Lenguaje Cealca, Caracas, Venezuela

Hospital de Clínicas Caracas, Caracas, Venezuela

S. Das
Technical University of Denmark, Kongens Lyngby, Denmark

Pioneer Centre for Artificial Intelligence, Copenhagen, Denmark
e-mail: sned@dtu.dk

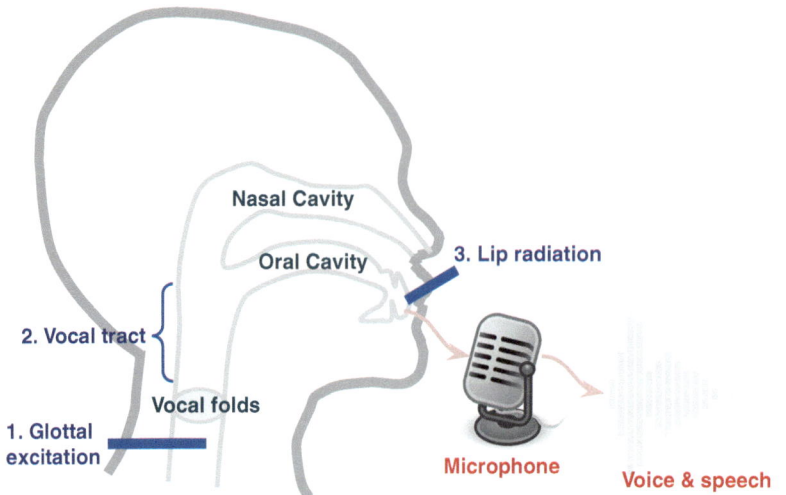

Fig. 5.1 Production of speech based on the source–filter model consisting of three parts (glottal excitation, vocal tract, and lip radiation). The source–filter model forms the basis for GIF. Human head adapted from https://commons.wikimedia.org/wiki/File:Source-filter_model_diagram.svg with licence CC-BY-SA-4.0

filters, which are adapted over short time frames (e.g. 30 ms). The key challenge is to model the frequency response of the vocal tract, whereas the lip radiation effect (i.e. conversion of flow at the lips into pressure in the free field) is typically modelled by a fixed high-pass filter. In most GIF methods, the estimation of the vocal tract and lip radiation can be computed automatically solely from the acoustic speech pressure signal recorded by a free-field microphone, which makes GIF analysis fully noninvasive. The use of the free-field microphone input enables applying inverse filtering in biomarking speakers' state of health from speech recordings conducted in real-life situations.

GIF provides a noninvasive method to estimate the origin of voiced speech, the glottal flow. Therefore, GIF reveals valuable information about phonation (e.g. fundamental frequency (F0) and phonation type) that is valuable in fundamental research on speech communication. Unlike a few other voice analysis techniques (such as electroglottography), GIF estimates a real acoustic phenomenon (airflow) that occurs in the human speech production mechanism. In addition, GIF can be used in technical applications, such as in the automatic speech-based classification of disorders and in speech synthesis.

GIF is an estimation method that, unfortunately, may sometimes show poor performance in the estimation of the glottal flow waveform. In particular, the accuracy of GIF is typically lower for high-pitched speech compared to low-pitched or medium-pitched speech. This decrease in estimation accuracy is due to problems in

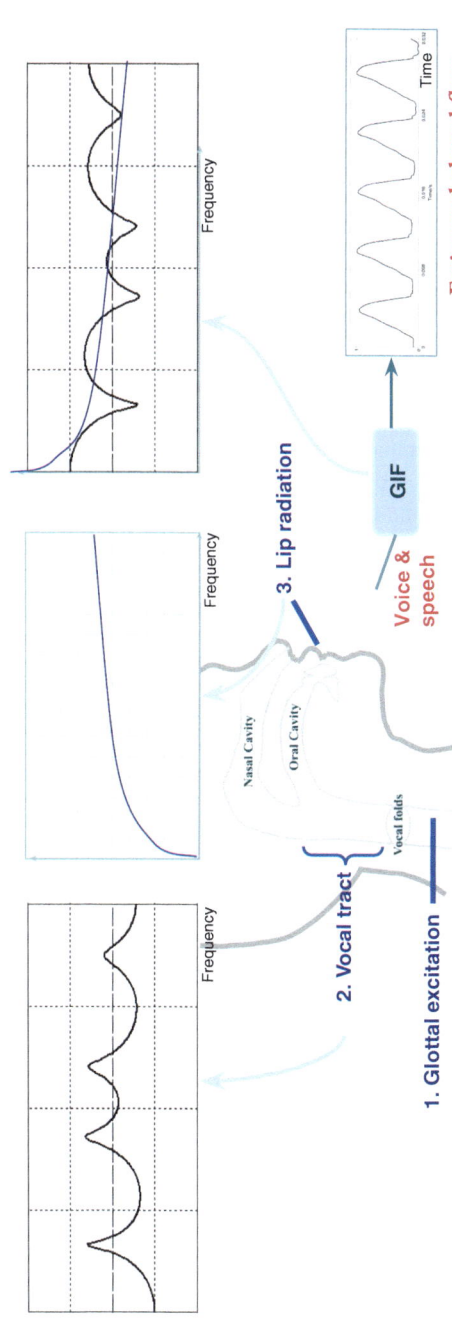

Fig. 5.2 The principle of GIF based on the source–filter model shown in Fig. 5.1. The speech signal recorded by a microphone is fed as input to GIF, which cancels the effects of the vocal tract and lip radiation. GIF provides an estimate of the glottal flow as output. Adapted from https://commons.wikimedia.org/wiki/File:Source-filter_model_diagram.svg with licence CC-BY-SA-4.0

the separation of the voice source and vocal tract from speech signals of high F0 [1]. The estimation of the first formant (F1) of the vocal tract is particularly vulnerable to the biasing effect caused by F0 and its lowest harmonics [2]. In addition, some GIF methods need user adjustments, which may result in the estimation results being biased by the user. An additional drawback of GIF is its vulnerability to the (technical) quality of the recording equipment. In particular, if the input speech signal is recorded using a microphone whose amplitude and phase responses are poor, the time-domain waveform of the estimated glottal flow will be distorted. To avoid such distortion, one should always use a high-quality omnidirectional condenser microphone in the recording of speech for GIF analysis. Finally, one should keep in mind that the simple linear source–tract model, which is used as the fundamental building block in most GIF methods, is unable to take into account nonlinear phenomena in speech production (e.g. interaction between source and tract). Therefore, one should not use GIF in studying nonlinear phenomena of speech production.

Voice source analysis is typically conducted in two stages. The first stage is GIF analysis, which takes as input the speech pressure signal recorded by a microphone and provides as output the time-domain waveform of the estimated glottal excitation. The second stage is the parameterization of the estimated glottal flow waveform. The output of the parameterization stage is a set of numerical values, glottal parameters that capture the most essential information embedded in the estimated time-domain glottal excitation waveform. Since both stages can be computed automatically (at least for most GIF methods), the combination of the two stages constitutes a pipeline with which a recorded speech signal can be converted into a single or a few numerical parameters to effectively model voice source information embedded in the speech signal.

5.2 Glottal Inverse Filtering Methods and Glottal Parameters

5.2.1 Glottal Inverse Filtering Methods

The idea of GIF was proposed by Miller [3], who used analogue inverse filters in his GIF implementation. Examples of other early studies based on analogue techniques are the studies conducted by Fant [4] and Lindqvist-Gauffin [5]. Rothenberg [2] introduced an analogue GIF method based on inverse filtering the volume velocity waveform recorded in the oral cavity instead of the speech pressure signal recorded in the free field outside the mouth. Rothenberg designed a special pneumotachograph mask, later referred to widely as Rothenberg's mask, which is a transducer capable of measuring the volume velocity at the mouth. The first GIF experiments based on digital signal processing were conducted independently of each other by Oppenheim and Schafer [6] as well as Nakatsui and Suzuki [7]. All GIF methods that have been proposed since the late 1970s are based on digital signal processing. Over the past four decades, many varying algorithms have been published, and some of them are listed below. Many of these methods (not necessarily all) use some form of linear prediction (LP) as a tool to compute a digital inverse model for the vocal tract. The use of LP introduces a remarkable improvement compared to older analogue GIF methods because the model adjusts automatically to the underlying speech signal without clumsy manual adjustments of analogue antiresonances.

- Closed phase analysis [8, 9].
- Iterative adaptive inverse filtering (IAIF) [10].
- Simultaneous inverse filtering and model matching [11]
- Zeros of Z-transform [12].
- Autoregressive model with an exogenous input [13].
- Complex cepstrum-based decomposition [14]
- Quasi-closed phase analysis [15]
- State-space modelling optimized by Kalman filtering [16, 17] or the expectation maximization algorithm [18].
- Quadratic programming [19].
- Modified IAIF [20].
- Deep neural network–based analysis [21, 22].
- Novel weighted LP and correntropy-based LP [23, 24].

5.2.2 Glottal Parameters

When a GIF is used in speech analysis, the obtained glottal flow waveforms need to be expressed in a parametric form in order to capture the most essential information embedded in the obtained time-domain waveforms. To parameterize glottal flow signals (or their first time-derivatives), several glottal parameters have been developed. They have been previously used mainly in the fundamental research of voice production, but recently also in modern machine learning (ML)-based classification studies on pathological voice (as will be described later in Sect. 5.4). Examples of common time-domain glottal parameters (see Figs. 5.3 and 5.4) are the open quotient, speed quotient, and closing quotient [25, 26], as well as the normalized amplitude quotient [27]. Examples of frequency-domain glottal parameters (see Fig. 5.5) are the level difference between the first and second harmonics (H1–H2) [28], harmonic richness factor [29], and parabolic spectral parameter [30].

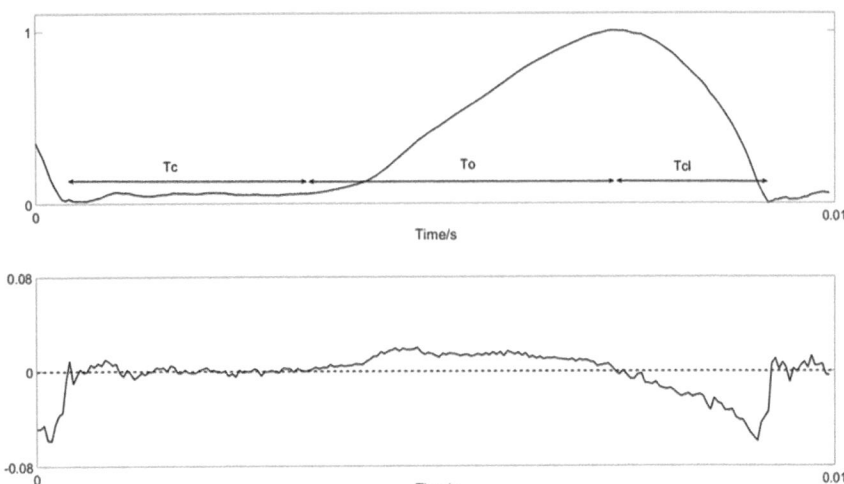

Fig. 5.3 Glottal pulse. An example of a glottal pulse (upper panel) and its derivative (lower panel) computed by GIF. Both waveforms are presented on an arbitrary amplitude scale. The glottal closed phase, opening phase, and closing phase are marked respectively by Tc, To, and Tcl. Time-domain glottal parameters can be computed from the marked time durations. As an example, the closing quotient can be computed as ClQ = Tcl/(Tc + To + Tcl)

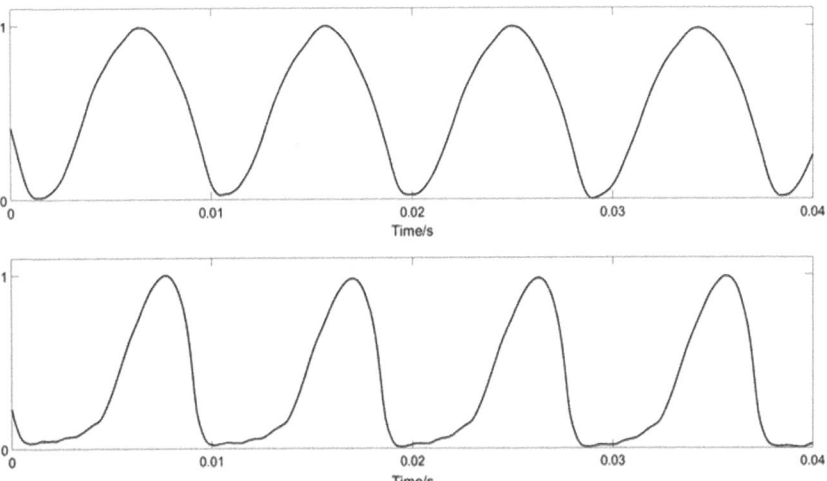

Fig. 5.4 Time-domain glottal flow pulse forms. Examples of time-domain glottal flow pulse forms computed by GIF from vowels produced using breathy phonation (upper panel) and pressed phonation (lower panel). The waveforms are presented on an arbitrary amplitude scale

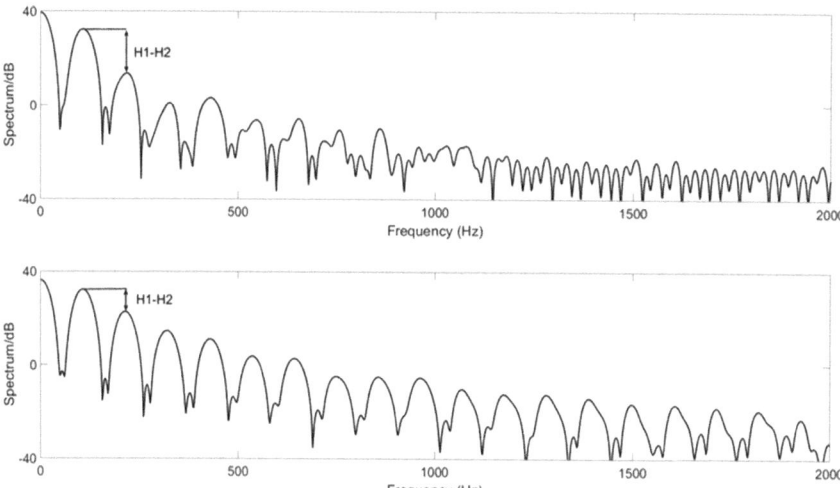

Fig. 5.5 Spectra of the glottal flow pulses shown in Fig. 5.4 in breathy phonation (upper panel) and in pressed phonation (lower panel). For visual clarity, the spectra are shown between 0 Hz and 2 kHz. The difference in spectral decay between the pulses is quantified by H1–H2. The value of H1–H2 is 18.4 dB and 9.6 dB in breathy and pressed phonation, respectively

5.3 Automatic Biomarking of Health from Voice

The main role of voice is to enable communication between people by transferring information between speakers. However, in addition to its linguistic content, speech also includes plenty of other content, such as paralinguistic information (e.g. vocal emotions such as sad vs. happy speech) and extralinguistic information (e.g. gender, age, and state of health of the speaker). A research question of increasing interest that takes advantage of extralinguistic acoustic cues of speech is posed by the following problem: Can we build a machine to automatically classify a human being's state of health using the person's voice signal? In the current article, this research topic is referred to as speech-based biomarking of health.

Speech-based biomarking of health benefits from the following issues. (1) Speech is a modality that is used by (almost) all the world's people as the main means of communication in everyday life. In addition, speech can be recorded today in a non-invasive and comfortable manner using a cost-effective device (e.g. a phone). Taken together, these two issues imply that speech constitutes a highly attractive and effective channel to biomark the state of health for a vast number of people all over the world. (2) Speech-based biomarking can be conducted outside the hospital, using a system that is economical, easy to administer, and capable of use by the patient at home, thereby avoiding frequent and often inconvenient visits to the clinic.

It is worth emphasizing that speech-based biomarking of health does not 'cure' the patient and does not replace true clinical diagnosis. Instead, the topic should be regarded as a potential preventive healthcare technology to detect diseases at an early stage, as well as track physiological changes caused by the disease. This issue is particularly useful, for example, in efforts to tackle neurodegenerative diseases (such as Parkinson's and Alzheimer's), which have become serious global health problems due to the ageing of populations. Particularly in neurodegenerative diseases, speech-based biomarking of health could, in principle, be used for the early detection of the disease even from telephone speech recordings.

Research in the automatic speech-based biomarking of health has expanded in the past five years. The topic relies heavily on ML and deep learning (DL) methodologies, but the role of signal processing is also important, particularly in converting speech signals to parametric feature vectors. The topic has been mainly studied from the point of view of the following two tasks. (1) The binary classification task (also known as the detection task). In this task, the machine aims to detect speakers with a certain disease (e.g. Parkinson's disease, heart failure, or COVID-19) from healthy controls. Today, the binary classification problem is by far the most widely studied topic in the area of speech-based biomarking of health. (2) The multi-class classification task. In this task, the machine aims to classify speech samples produced by speakers suffering from various diseases (e.g. healthy vs. hyperfunctional dysphonia vs. vocal fold paresis) or to classify speakers with differing disease severity levels (e.g. healthy vs. mild dysarthria vs. severe dysarthria).

In this article, we will focus on the detection task. Two technologies (the classical pipeline approach and the end-to-end approach) are first generally described in this section. Then we describe two examples of our own studies where the automatic speech-based detection of diseases has been investigated using GIF.

The Classical Pipeline Approach: Figure 5.6 shows a general flow diagram of an ML-based classifier system that detects a disease (named "X") from speech. It is worth noting that this diagram (due to the use of ML) consists of the system training and testing parts, which are shown, respectively, by the upper and lower parts of

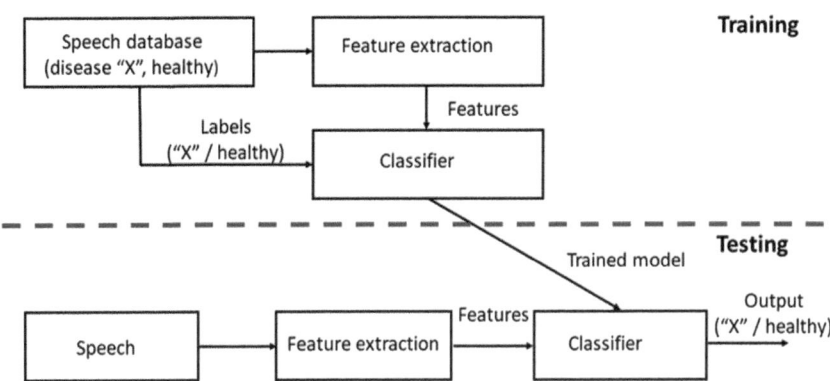

Fig. 5.6 Block diagram of a detection system. A general block diagram of a detection system based on the classical pipeline approach. The speech database includes labelled speech signals (disease "X" vs. healthy). The classifier can be, for example, a Support Vector Machine (SVM)

Fig. 5.6. The system architecture is called the classical pipeline because it consists of two separate components, the feature extraction stage and the classifier stage. The system is built based on supervised learning, in which the second key component of the system, the classifier, is first trained with labelled speech data in the training phase. The training of the classifier is performed by first presenting speech using a compressed set of preselected features. There are numerous different features available today, and new features are still being developed in the study area. An example of a widely used feature is the mel-frequency cepstral coefficient (MFCC) set [31]. There are also many possible classifiers to be used in the study area. One of the most widely used classifiers is the support vector machine (SVM) [32].

Figure 5.7 shows a simplified example, which visualizes how the SMV classifier has learned in the training phase to distinguish speech samples of the two classes shown in Fig. 5.6. In the test phase (which is also known as the inference phase), the speech signal, which is to be automatically classified, is first converted into features using the same feature extraction method that was used in the training phase. The final decision (i.e. "healthy" vs. "disease X") is made by the trained classifier based on the decision boundary, which the classifier learned in the training phase. Because the two classes in the original, low-dimensional feature space are not necessarily linearly separable, SVM implicitly maps the data to a higher-dimensional space using a kernel function.

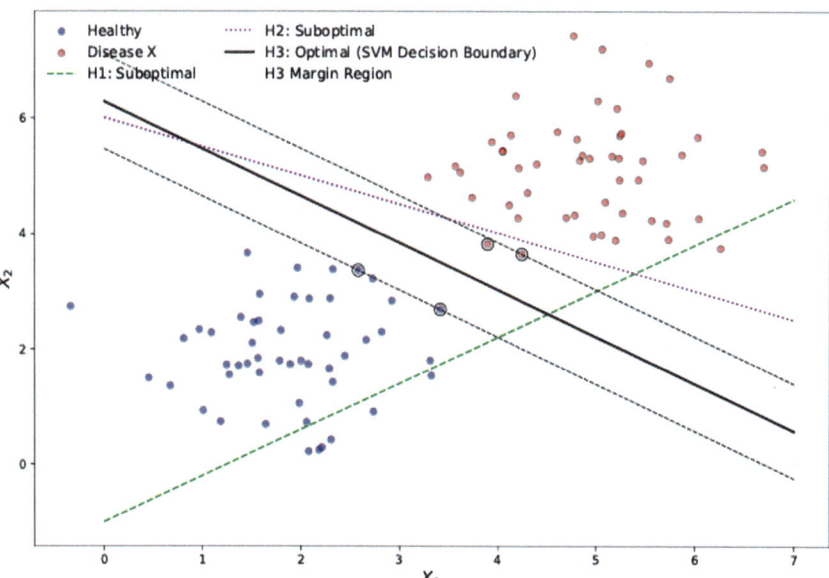

Fig. 5.7 Training data. A simplified example showing training data in two classes (red circles: "Disease X"; blue circles: "Healthy") in a 2-dimensional speech feature space. In the training phase, SVM defines the decision boundary (H3), which separates the classes with the maximal margin. Test samples are mapped into that same space, and they are finally classified either as "Healthy" or "Disease X," based on the side of the decision boundary where they fall

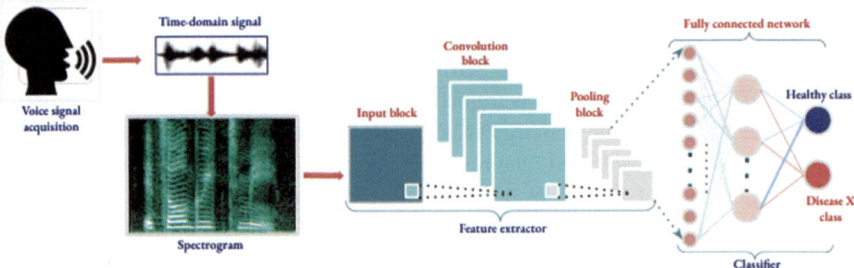

Fig. 5.8 CNN-based end-to-end classification system. An example of a CNN-based end-to-end classification system (binary detection between "disease X" and "healthy" voice)

The End-to-End Approach Rapid technological development in the past few years has made it possible to use classifiers that classify speech directly from the time-domain raw waveform (or from a spectrogram) instead of using pre-selected features and a separate classifier stage as in the classical pipeline approach shown in Fig. 5.6. These modern classifiers are called end-to-end classifiers. They are typically built using a structure that consists of many neural network layers. A popular classifier used in this area is the convolutional neural net (CNN) shown in Fig. 5.8. End-to-end systems do not have a separate feature extraction stage, but the system consists of a single network structure, which is trained as a whole. In the testing phase, the raw input speech signal (or its spectrogram) is filtered with the trained network whose last layer gives the predicted class (e.g. "healthy" vs. "pathological" in Fig. 5.8) as output. It is worth emphasizing that DL-based end-to-end classifiers call for larger amounts of training data compared to classical pipeline systems. In speech-based biomarking of health, the volume of training data is, however, typically small, and therefore classical ML-based pipeline systems may provide better classification performance than modern DL-based end-to-end systems.

5.4 Machine Learning Studies in the Automatic Classification of Diseases Using Glottal Inverse Filtering

Automatic speech-based biomarking of diseases (particularly Parkinson's disease) has been studied widely in recent years. The studies conducted have mainly used the classical pipeline architecture, but recently also the CNN-based end-to-end architecture. For the pipeline systems, many different ML classifiers as well as various existing feature sets have been used. For more information about different kinds of features and classifiers used in the speech-based biomarking of health, the reader is referred to the reviews published in [33–35]. In some biomarking studies, glottal features based on GIF have been used in feature extraction. Examples of studies where glottal features have been used in the automatic speech-based detection of diseases are given below:

- Classification of vocal nodules in children [36–38].
- Pathology classification [39–42].
- Detection of Parkinson's disease [43–47].
- Intelligibility assessment of dysarthric speech [48].
- Detection of Covid-19 [49].
- Detection of depression [50, 51].

Next, we will describe in more detail two of our own studies on automatic detection of disorders from speech, where ML and DL classifiers have been trained using glottal features computed using GIF.

In [52], we published an article on speech-based biomarking of heart failure (HF), which is one of the first studies on the automatic detection of HF. The study used a smallish Finnish database of speech produced by 20 HF patients and 25 healthy controls. The patients were hospitalized for HF of any aetiology, either due to acute symptom worsening or for diagnostic tests related to advanced HF. We built various classical pipeline systems using four classifiers (SVM, Extra Tree (ET), AdaBoost, and feed-forward neural network (FFNN)) and two individual feature sets (MFCCs and glottal features). In addition, we evaluated the classifiers by combining the two feature sets as well as by using a feature selection algorithm. The main results of the study are shown in terms of accuracy in Table 5.1. The results show that the best system (based on the FFNN classifier and the combination of the MFCC and glottal features) gave an accuracy of about 82%. This result shows that the glottal features include useful voice source information, which is not represented adequately by the MFCC features. Therefore, complementing the MFCC features with the glottal features helps the machine in the detection task. We argue that one possible reason why better voice source information aided the machine in the detection task could be the generation of oedema at the vocal folds in HF. Generation of oedema may have changed the characteristics of the glottal flow for the HF patients. This possible explanation is demonstrated in Fig. 5.9, which shows examples of estimated glottal flows computed from the voices of a healthy speaker and an HF patient. The figure shows that the general shape of the glottal flow pulse is smoother (i.e. breathier) for the HF patient compared to the healthy speaker.

Table 5.1 Classification accuracy

Classifier	MFS (104)	GFS (192)	MFS + GFS (296)	MFS + GFS with feature selection (85)
SVM	76.26	65.59	75.52	77.15
ET	68.07	64.15	64.8	72.29
AdaBoost	76.54	68.85	73.04	79.23
FFNN	77.02	71.03	75.34	81.51

Classification accuracy (in %) for the four classifiers and four feature sets studied in [52]. MFS: the mel-frequency cepstral coefficient set; GFS: the glottal feature set. The feature dimension is given in parentheses

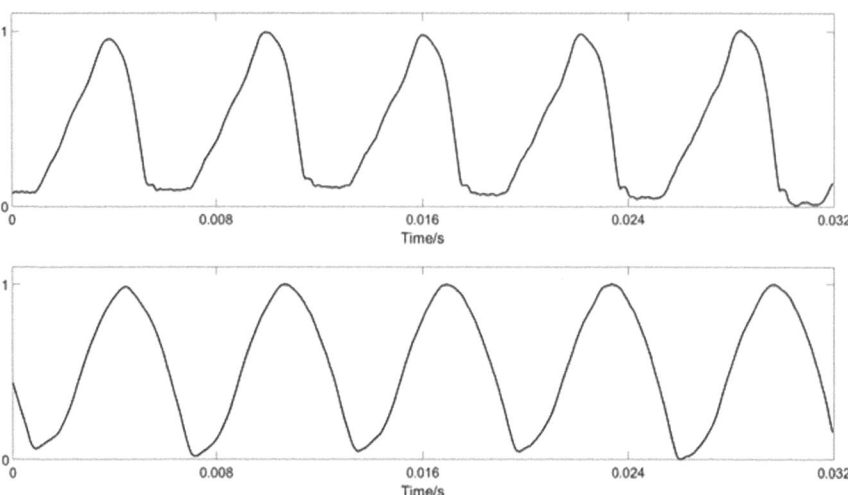

Fig. 5.9 Glottal flow signals. Examples of glottal flow signals estimated by GIF from the healthy and pathological speech studied in [52]. The upper shows a flow signal estimated from a vowel produced by a healthy male speaker. The lower panel shows a flow signal estimated from a vowel produced by a male heart failure patient. The waveforms are presented on an arbitrary amplitude scale

The second example is our study published in [53] on the detection of dysarthric and dysphonic voices. The dysarthric voices were produced by speakers with Amyotrophic Lateral Sclerosis (ALS) and Cerebral Palsy (CP), and the speech data was taken from two open databases (UA-Speech [54] and TORGO [55]). The dysphonic samples were taken from the open UPM database [56, 57]. For the detection of both pathologies, we built two types of detection systems (classical pipeline systems and end-to-end systems) by using glottal flow waveforms estimated by GIF and glottal parameters. For the classical pipeline approach, we used the SVM classifier and compared two general speech feature sets, referred to as openSMILE-1 and openSMILE-2 in [53], and two glottal feature sets, referred to as Glottal-1 and Glottal-2 in [53] (for more details, see Section II.B in [53]). For the end-to-end approach, we built a system consisting of multiple layers of CNN followed by a multilayer perceptron. For this system, we compared two types of time-domain raw waveform input: the speech pressure signal (which is the default choice for the raw waveform input in end-to-end systems) and the glottal flow, which was estimated using GIF. As the GIF algorithm, we use the quasi-closed phase (QCP) method [15]. The results of the detection experiments obtained using the classical pipeline approach are shown in Table 5.2 for all three databases and for all feature sets. The general trend of the results indicates that the best results were obtained when the glottal features were combined with the baseline openSMILE features. The results obtained for the end-to-end systems shown in Table 5.3 indicate higher accuracies (about 2–3% absolute improvement in all three databases) when glottal flow was used as the raw time-domain input, compared to using the default raw input, the

5 Glottal Inverse Filtering and Its Application in the Automatic Classification...

Table 5.2 Classification results with classical pipeline architecture

Feature set	UA-Speech			TORGO			UPM		
	Accuracy (%)	Sensitivity (%)	Specificity (%)	Accuracy (%)	Sensitivity (%)	Specificity (%)	Accuracy (%)	Sensitivity (%)	Specificity (%)
OpenSMILE-1	76.65	73.76	79.54	78.24	72.94	83.54	70.73	78.49	62.98
OpenSMILE-2	86.99	82.35	91.63	80.62	73.73	87.52	72.50	77.61	67.84
Glottal-1	73.56	76.47	70.65	67.17	71.22	63.12	63.17	67.08	59.27
Glottal-2	68.74	69.36	68.12	66.93	71.55	62.17	64.63	65.85	63.41
OpenSMILE-1 + Glottal-1	81.01	82.55	79.48	79.62	73.21	86.03	73.39	79.54	67.24
OpenSMILE-2 + Glottal-1	91.88	92.56	91.21	82.12	79.02	85.22	75.61	79.11	72.20
OpenSMILE-1 + Glottal-2	80.02	81.93	78.12	80.63	72.59	88.68	74.17	80.05	68.29
OpenSMILE-2 + Glottal-2	91.19	91.57	90.82	81.35	76.83	85.87	76.83	80.81	73.36

Classification results (in %) obtained in [53] using the classical pipeline architecture based on the SVM classifier. Results are shown for the different openS-MILE and glottal features and for the three pathological voice databases studied

Table 5.3 Classification results with the end-to-end

Network	Input	UA-Speech			TORGO			UPM		
		Accuracy (%)	Sensitivity (%)	Specificity (%)	Accuracy (%)	Sensitivity (%)	Specificity (%)	Accuracy (%)	Sensitivity (%)	Specificity (%)
CNN+MLP	Raw speech	85.12	80.85	89.40	78.83	82.85	76.24	73.71	75.92	71.35
	Glottal flow	87.93	86.65	90.62	81.12	85.88	75.26	76.66	80.50	73.50
CNN+LSTM	Raw speech	74.19	69.26	81.48	71.15	78.45	66.17	63.24	65.53	59.92
	Glottal flow	77.57	73.13	82.48	75.41	81.32	69.68	72.22	76.56	68.14

Classification results (in %) obtained using the end-to-end architecture for the three pathological voice databases studied in [53]

speech waveform. Taken together, the study showed that the usage of glottal source information (estimated by GIF) helped to improve the automatic detection of pathological voice, both for classical pipeline systems and for end-to-end systems.

5.5 Summary and Conclusions

Glottal inverse filtering (GIF) is a voice source analysis method that enables noninvasive estimation of the voice source from microphone speech signals. Many GIF methods and glottal parameters have been developed during the past five decades, and new GIF methods have been proposed recently. GIF has been mainly used in the fundamental research of speech and singing to study voice source characteristics, for example, in intensity regulation [58, 59], voice quality and vocal emotions [60, 61], as well as the range of singing styles [62, 63]. In recent years, GIF has also been used with ML and DL classifiers in speech-based biomarking of health. In this application area, GIF is typically used in classical pipeline classifiers to extract features that carry voice source information. In addition, the estimated glottal flow waveforms can be used in end-to-end classifiers as an alternative raw time-domain input to the speech signal.

Using glottal features together with widely used speech features (e.g. MFCCs [31], openSMILE [37]) has been shown to improve detection accuracy in several of our recent biomarker studies (e.g. [41, 47, 53, 64]). In other words, the utilization of glottal features per se is not necessarily the best way to extract features for the automatic classification of diseases. However, glottal features convey complementary information about the voice source that is not necessarily adequately represented by the popular feature sets, which are used in speech-based biomarking studies. Therefore, combining glottal features with existing speech feature sets has mostly turned out to be the best feature extraction strategy in our biomarking studies.

In speech-based biomarking of health, DL-based end-to-end approaches are becoming popular today. Since voice source information is embedded in the speech signal, this information could, in principle, be extracted by nonlinear end-to-end networks without using GIF as a preprocessing stage to compute glottal features. However, end-to-end networks are data-hungry, and they cannot necessarily be trained properly in the study area of pathological voice, where only small amounts of training data are typically available. Therefore, it is still justified to use classical pipeline systems in which glottal features are combined with other known speech feature sets to better model voice source information. In addition, the utilization of glottal features in modern speech-based health applications is beneficial for clinicians because these features have better explainability compared to DL-based end-to-end systems, which, unfortunately, are "black boxes" that hide their internal logic from the user.

References

1. Alku P. Glottal inverse filtering analysis of human voice production. A review of estimation and parameterization methods of the glottal excitation and their applications. Sādhanā. 2011;36(5):623–50. https://doi.org/10.1007/s12046-011-0041.
2. Rothenberg M. A new inverse-filtering technique for deriving the glottal air flow waveform during voicing. J Acoust Soc Am. 1973;53(6):1632–45. https://doi.org/10.1121/1.1913513.
3. Miller RL. Nature of the vocal cord wave. J Acoust Soc Am. 1959;31(6):667–77. https://doi.org/10.1121/1.1907771.
4. Fant G. A new anti-resonance circuit for inverse filtering. Speech Transm Lab Q Prog Status Rep. 1961;2(1):1–6.
5. Lindqvist-Gauffin J. Studies of the voice source by means of inverse filtering. Speech Transm Lab Q Prog Status Rep. 1965;6(1):8–13.
6. Oppenheim A, Schafer R. Homomorphic analysis of speech. IEEE Trans Audio Electroacoust. 1968;16:221–6. https://doi.org/10.1109/tau.1968.1161965.
7. Nakatsui M, Suzuki J. Method of observation of glottal-source wave using digital inverse filtering in time domain. J Acoust Soc Am. 1970;1(47):664–5.
8. Strube HW. Determination of the instant of glottal closure from the speech wave. J Acoust Soc Am. 1974;56(5):1625–9.
9. Wong D, Markel J, Gray A. Least squares glottal inverse filtering from the acoustic speech waveform. IEEE Trans Acoust Speech Signal Process. 1979;27:350–5.
10. Alku P. Glottal wave analysis with pitch synchronous iterative adaptive inverse filtering. Speech Commun. 1992;11(2–3):109–18.
11. Fröhlich M, Michaelis D, Strube HW. SIM – simultaneous inverse filtering and matching of a glottal flow model for acoustic speech signals. J Acoust Soc Am. 2001;110(1):479–88. https://doi.org/10.1121/1.1379076.
12. Bozkurt B, Doval B, d'Alessandro C, Dutoit T. Zeros of z-transform representation with application to source-filter separation in speech. IEEE Signal Process. Lett. 2005;12(4):344–7.
13. Fu Q, Murphy P. Robust glottal source estimation based on joint source-filter model optimization. IEEE Trans Audio Speech Lang Process. 2006;14(1):492–501.
14. Drugman T, Bozkurt B, Dutoit T. Causal–anticausal decomposition of speech using complex cepstrum for glottal source estimation. Speech Commun. 2011;53:855–66. https://doi.org/10.1016/j.specom.2011.02.004.
15. Airaksinen M, Raitio T, Story B, Alku P. Quasi closed phase glottal inverse filtering analysis with weighted linear prediction. IEEE Trans Audio Speech Lang Process. 2013;22(3):596–607. https://doi.org/10.1109/taslp.2013.2294585.
16. Sahoo S, Routray A. A novel method of glottal inverse filtering. IEEE Trans Audio Speech Lang Process. 2016;24(7):1230–41. https://doi.org/10.1109/taslp.2016.2551864.
17. Cortés JP, Alzamendi GA, Weinstein AJ, Yuz JI, Espinoza VM, Mehta DD, et al. Kalman filter implementation of subglottal impedance-based inverse filtering to estimate glottal airflow during phonation. Appl Sci. 2021;12(1):401. https://doi.org/10.3390/app12010401.
18. Alzamendi GA, Schlotthauer G. Modeling and joint estimation of glottal source and vocal tract filter by state-space methods. Biomed Signal Process Control. 2017;37:5–15. https://doi.org/10.1016/j.bspc.2016.12.022.
19. Airaksinen M, Backstrom T, Alku P. Quadratic programming approach to glottal inverse filtering by joint norm-1 and norm-2 optimization. IEEE Trans Audio Speech Lang Process. 2016;25(5):929–39. https://doi.org/10.1109/taslp.2016.2620718.
20. Mokhtari P, Story B, Alku P, Ando H. Estimation of the glottal flow from speech pressure signals: evaluation of three variants of iterative adaptive inverse filtering using computational physical modelling of voice production. Speech Commun. 2018;12(104):24–38. https://doi.org/10.1016/j.specom.2018.09.005.
21. Narendra NP, Airaksinen M, Story B, Alku P. Estimation of the glottal source from coded telephone speech using deep neural networks. Speech Commun. 2019;106:95–104.

22. Langheinrich I, Stone S, Zhang X, Birkholz P. Glottal inverse filtering based on articulatory synthesis and deep learning. Proc Interspeech. 2022:1327–31.
23. Zalazar IA, Alzamendi GA, Schlotthauer G. Symmetric and asymmetric Gaussian weighted linear prediction for voice inverse filtering. Speech Commun. 2024;159:103057. https://doi.org/10.1016/j.specom.2024.103057.
24. Zalazar IA, Alzamendi GA, Zañartu M, Schlotthauer G. Correntropy-based linear prediction for voice inverse filtering. In: Proceedings of the 18th international symposium on medical information processing and analysis, vol. 12567. SPIE; 2023. p. 356–65. https://doi.org/10.1117/12.2669810.
25. Timcke R, von Leden H, Moore P. Laryngeal vibrations: measurements of the glottic wave. Archiv Otolaryngol. 1958;68(1):1–9.
26. Monsen RB, Engebretson AM. Study of variations in the male and female glottal wave. J Acoust Soc Am. 1977;62(4):981–93.
27. Alku P, Bäckström T, Vilkman E. Normalized amplitude quotient for parametrization of the glottal flow. J Acoust Soc Am. 2002;112(2):701–10. https://doi.org/10.1121/1.1490365.
28. Titze IR, Sundberg J. Vocal intensity in speakers and singers. J Acoust Soc Am. 1992;91(5):2936–46. https://doi.org/10.1121/1.402929.
29. Childers DG, Lee CK. Vocal quality factors: analysis, synthesis, and perception. J Acoust Soc Am. 1991;90(5):2394–410. https://doi.org/10.1121/1.402044.
30. Alku P, Strik H, Vilkman E. Parabolic spectral parameter – a new method for quantification of the glottal flow. Speech Commun. 1997;22(1):67–79. https://doi.org/10.1016/S0167-6393(97)00020-4.
31. Davis S, Mermelstein P. Comparison of parametric representations for monosyllabic word recognition in continuously spoken sentences. IEEE Trans Acoust Speech Signal Process. 1980;28(4):357–66.
32. Cortes C, Vapnik V. Support-vector networks, Mach Learn 20 1995;(3): 273-297. doi: https://doi.org/10.1007/BF00994018
33. Cummins N, Baird A, Schuller BW. Speech analysis for health: current state-of-the-art and the increasing impact of deep learning. Methods. 2018;151:41–54. https://doi.org/10.1016/j.ymeth.2018.07.007.
34. Moro-Velazquez L, Gomez-Garcia JA, Arias-Londoño JD, Dehak N, Godino-Llorente JI. Advances in Parkinson's Disease detection and assessment using voice and speech: a review of the articulatory and phonatory aspects. Biomed Sig Process Control. 2021;66:102418. https://doi.org/10.1016/j.bspc.2021.102418.
35. Hecker P, Steckhan N, Eyben F, Schuller BW, Arnrich B. Voice analysis for neurological disorder recognition – a systematic review and perspective on emerging trends. Front Digit Health. 2022;4:842301. https://doi.org/10.3389/fdgth.2022.842301.
36. Kaushik M, Baghel N, Burget R, Travieso CM, Dutta MK. SLINet: dysphasia detection in children using deep neural network. Biomed Signal Process Control. 2021;68:102798.
37. Eyben F, Wöllmer M, Schuller B. Opensmile: the Munich versatile and fast open-source audio feature extractor. Proc ACM Int Conf Multimedia. 2010:1459–62.
38. Szklanny K, Wrzeciono P. The application of a genetic algorithm in the noninvasive assessment of vocal nodules in children. IEEE Access. 2019;7:44966–76. https://doi.org/10.1109/access.2019.2908313.
39. Wu Y, Zhou C, Fan Z, Wu D, Zhang X, Tao Z. Investigation and evaluation of glottal flow waveform for voice pathology detection. IEEE Access. 2020;9:30–44. https://doi.org/10.1109/access.2020.3046767.
40. Gómez-Vilda P, Fernández-Baillo R, Rodellar-Biarge V, Lluis VN, Álvarez-Marquina A, Mazaira-Fernández LM, et al. Glottal Source biometrical signature for voice pathology detection. Speech Commun. 2008;51(9):759–81. https://doi.org/10.1016/j.specom.2008.09.005.
41. Kadiri SR, Alku P. Analysis and detection of pathological voice using glottal source features. IEEE J Sel Top Signal Process. 2019;14(2):367–79. https://doi.org/10.48550/arXiv.2309.14080.

42. Tirronen S, Kadiri SR, Alku P. Hierarchical multi-class classification of voice disorders using self-supervised models and glottal features. IEEE Open J Signal Process. 2023;4:80–8. https://doi.org/10.1109/OJSP.2023.3242862.
43. Novotný M, Dušek P, Daly I, Růžička E, Rusz J. Glottal source analysis of voice deficits in newly diagnosed drug-naïve patients with Parkinson's disease: correlation between acoustic speech characteristics and non-speech motor performance. Biomed Signal Process Control. 2020;57:101818. https://doi.org/10.1016/j.bspc.2019.101818.
44. Vásquez-Correa JC, Fritsch J, Orozco-Arroyave JR, Nöth E, Magimai-Doss M. On modeling glottal source information for phonation assessment in Parkinson's disease. Proc Interspeech. 2021:26–30. https://doi.org/10.21437/Interspeech.2021-1084.
45. Narendra NP, Schuller B, Alku P. The detection of Parkinson's disease from speech using voice source information. IEEE Trans Audio Speech Lang Process. 2021;29:1925–36. https://doi.org/10.1109/TASLP.2021.3078364.
46. Reddy MK, Alku P. Exemplar-based sparse representations for detection of Parkinson's disease from speech. IEEE/ACM Trans Audio Speech Lang Process. 2023;31:1386–96. https://doi.org/10.1109/TASLP.2023.3260709.
47. Liu Y, Reddy MK, Penttilä N, Ihalainen T, Alku P, Räsänen O. Automatic assessment of Parkinson's disease using speech representations of phonation and articulation. IEEE/ACM Trans Audio Speech Lang Process. 2022;31:242–55. https://doi.org/10.1109/TASLP.2022.3212829.
48. Narendra NP, Alku P. Automatic intelligibility assessment of dysarthric speech using glottal parameters. Speech Commun. 2020;123:1–9. https://doi.org/10.1016/j.specom.2020.06.003.
49. Deshmukh S, Al Ismail M, Singh R. Interpreting glottal flow dynamics for detecting covid-19 from voice. Proc Icassp. 2021:1055–9. https://doi.org/10.1109/ICASSP39728.2021.9414530.
50. Ooi KE, Low LS, Lech M, Allen N. Early prediction of major depression in adolescents using glottal wave characteristics and teager energy parameters. Proc Icassp. 2012:4613–6. https://doi.org/10.1109/ICASSP.2012.6288946.
51. Simantiraki O, Charonyktakis P, Pampouchidou A, Tsiknakis M, Cooke M. Glottal source features for automatic speech-based depression assessment. Proc Interspeech. 2017:2700–4. https://doi.org/10.21437/Interspeech.2017-1251.
52. Reddy MK, Helkkula P, Keerthana YM, Kaitue K, Minkkinen M, Tolppanen H, Nieminen T, Alku P. The automatic detection of heart failure using speech signals. Comp Speech Lang. 2021;69:101205. https://doi.org/10.1016/j.csl.2021.101205.
53. Hegde S, Shetty S, Rai S, Dodderi T. A survey on machine learning approaches for automatic detection of voice disorders. J Voice. 2019;33(6):947.e11–33. https://doi.org/10.1016/j.jvoice.2018.07.014.
54. Kim H, Hasegawa-Johnson M, Perlman A, Gunderson JR, Huang TS, Watkin KL, Frame S. Dysarthric speech database for universal access research. Proc Interspeech. 2008:1741–4. https://doi.org/10.21437/Interspeech.2008-480.
55. Rudzicz F, Namasivayam AK, Wolff T. The TORGO database of acoustic and articulatory speech from speakers with dysarthria. Lang Resour Eval. 2012;46:523–41. https://doi.org/10.1007/s10579-011-9145-0.
56. Moro-Velázquez L, Gómez-García JA, Godino-Llorente JI, Andrade-Miranda G. Modulation spectra morphological parameters: a new method to assess voice pathologies according to the GRBAS scale. Biomed Res Int. 2015;2015:259239. https://doi.org/10.1155/2015/259239.
57. Arias-Londoño JD, Godino-Llorente JI, Markaki M, Stylianou Y. On combining information from modulation spectra and mel-frequency cepstral coefficients for automatic detection of pathological voices. Logoped Phoniatr Vocol. 2011;36(2):60–9. https://doi.org/10.3109/14015439.2010.528788.
58. Alku P, Airas M, Björkner E, Sundberg J. An amplitude quotient based method to analyze changes in the shape of the glottal pulse in the regulation of vocal intensity. J Acoust Soc Am. 2006;120(2):1052–62. https://doi.org/10.1121/1.2211589.

59. Holmberg EB, Hillman RE, Perkell JS. Glottal airflow and transglottal air pressure measurements for male and female speakers in soft, normal, and loud voice. J Acoust Soc Am. 1988;84(2):511–29. https://doi.org/10.1121/1.396829.
60. Airas M, Alku P. Emotions in vowel segments of continuous speech: analysis of the glottal flow using the normalised amplitude quotient. Phonetica. 2006;63(1):26–46. https://doi.org/10.1159/000091405.
61. Gobl C, Chasaide AN. Acoustic characteristics of voice quality. Speech Commun. 1992;11(4-5):481–90. https://doi.org/10.1016/0167-6393(92)90055-C.
62. Sundberg J, Fahlstedt E, Morell A. Effects on the glottal voice source of vocal loudness variation in untrained female and male voices. J Acoust Soc Am. 2005;117(2):879–85. https://doi.org/10.1121/1.1841612.
63. Sundberg J, Titze I, Scherer R. Phonatory control in male singing: a study of the effects of subglottal pressure, fundamental frequency, and mode of phonation on the voice source. J Voice. 1993;7(1):15–29. https://doi.org/10.1016/s0892-1997(05)80108-0.
64. Reddy MK, Alku P. A comparison of cepstral features in the detection of pathological voices by varying the input and filterbank of the cepstrum computation. IEEE Access. 2021;9:135953–63. https://doi.org/10.1109/ACCESS.2021.3117665.

Open Access This chapter is licensed under the terms of the Creative Commons Attribution-NonCommercial-NoDerivatives 4.0 International License (http://creativecommons.org/licenses/by-nc-nd/4.0/), which permits any noncommercial use, sharing, distribution and reproduction in any medium or format, as long as you give appropriate credit to the original author(s) and the source, provide a link to the Creative Commons license and indicate if you modified the licensed material. You do not have permission under this license to share adapted material derived from this chapter or parts of it.

The images or other third party material in this chapter are included in the chapter's Creative Commons license, unless indicated otherwise in a credit line to the material. If material is not included in the chapter's Creative Commons license and your intended use is not permitted by statutory regulation or exceeds the permitted use, you will need to obtain permission directly from the copyright holder.

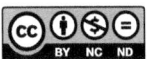

AI Models for Voice Disorders: Considerations from Development to Deployment

Sneha Das

Building Voice AI for pathology differs from conventional voice AI because (i) voice signals vary across languages, tasks, microphones and rooms, more so in pathological and clinical settings, *and* (ii) labelled clinical data are scarce and imbalanced, and (iii) clinical use demands interpretability, governance, and long-term maintenance. Through this chapter, we hope to provide an engineering roadmap that connects voice biomarker discovery to model design and, crucially, to deployment constraints in healthcare settings. Voice artificial intelligence (AI), refers to the broader domain of (semi) automated tools that work with voice and vocal sounds, including speech, as input. The tools map the input, a sound signal, to the target output. The target tasks associated with voice AI within vocal disorders and pathological voices range from objective screening aiding perceptual tests like the GRBAS tests to diagnosing voice cancer and neurodegenerative diseases and disorders [1, 2]. A typical voice AI is illustrated in Fig. 6.1 and coarsely comprises an input signal block, a model block that maps the input to useful representations, and an output block. The input block is a voice signal that is further preprocessed to convert into features. These features are closely associated with voice biomarkers, discussed in the previous chapters. The features are input to the models, ranging from classical statistical models to more advanced deep-learning and foundation models. The output of these models is the final desired outcome of the tool, like an outcome from screening for vocal cancer.

S. Das (✉)
Technical University of Denmark, Kongens Lyngby, Denmark

Pioneer Centre for Artificial Intelligence, Copenhagen, Denmark
e-mail: sned@dtu.dk

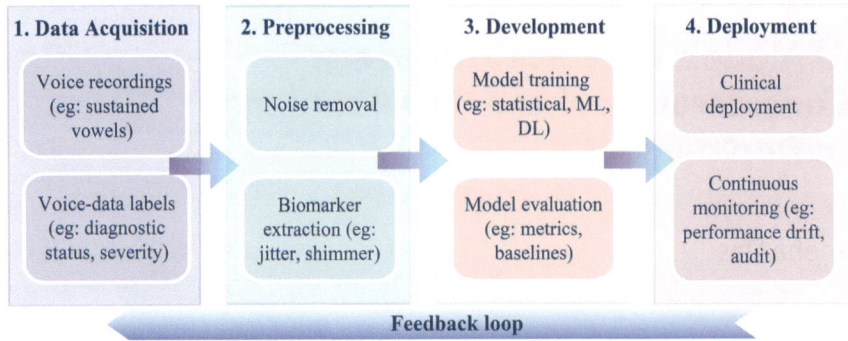

Fig. 6.1 Typical voice AI tool

6.1 Learning from Voice: Modeling Strategies Across Paradigms

Modelling in Voice AI translates measurable vocal biomarkers, like acoustic, prosodic, and spectral features, into diagnostic or prognostic outcomes. Depending on data scale, quality, and intended clinical use, models range from transparent statistical analyses to end-to-end neural systems. This section outlines these modeling families, their relative advantages, and their suitability for different stages of Voice AI development. A review of recent studies on Parkinson's disease detection from voice signals shows that most systems rely on traditional machine learning over hand-crafted acoustic features, while deep learning is gaining ground as datasets expand. The distribution presented in Fig. 6.2. The methods of modelling can thus be broadly divided into statistical modelling, machine learning, and deep learning. These categories are further discussed in the remaining part of the section, followed by a section on factors to consider when choosing an AI model and a brief introduction to foundation models and their potential for use within voice analysis.

6.1.1 The Modeling Spectrum in Voice AI

Statistical analysis is often the first step in Voice AI pipelines [3]. It is usually employed to investigate the correlation between candidate biomarkers and the target diagnostic outcomes or endpoints, aiding in the selection of relevant acoustic features and generating hypotheses. Statistical techniques like ANOVA, t-test and logistic regression quantify feature-outcome relations and provide directly interpretable coefficients and effect sizes. However, they assume linearity and independence, and thus are limited in modeling complex, nonlinear voice-disease dynamics. Their value lies in explainability and as an evidence base for subsequent machine learning.

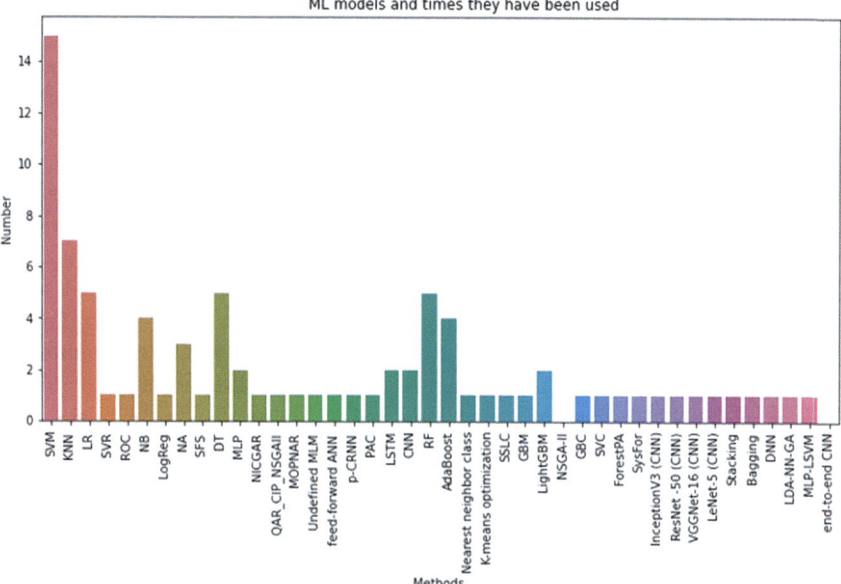

Fig. 6.2 Usage of ML Models. Distribution showing the different models. (Based on an overview of papers in collaboration with M. Pedersen)

Machine learning and deep learning. Voice AI has evolved from hand-crafted acoustic classifiers to models that learn directly from raw sound. In practice, these systems are framed as a) classification tasks: distinguishing, for instance, early and advanced Parkinson's disease from healthy controls, or as b) regression tasks predicting continuous severity scores. Classical machine-learning models such as support vector machines (SVMs), random forests, k-nearest neighbours, and regularized linear regression remain the workhorses of the field. They operate on engineered acoustic features or biomarkers, such as jitter, shimmer, formants, and spectral measures [2], acoustic features extracted from sustained vowels as input. These methods offer stable and consistent performance on small to medium datasets. Their relative transparency allows clinicians to trace which features contribute to a diagnostic outcome, making them particularly suitable for early-stage clinical prototypes or quality-control pipelines. Deep-learning architectures, including fully connected networks, convolutional neural networks (CNNs), recurrent or long short-term memory (LSTM) models, and the newer transformer-based systems, shift the paradigm by learning hierarchical representations directly from waveforms or spectrograms. These models capture complex, nonlinear relations in the signal that may correspond to pathological tremor, instability, or spectral noise patterns that are imperceptible to humans. However, their power comes at a cost: they require large, diverse datasets, strong regularization, and careful domain adaptation to generalize across recording conditions, languages, and devices. The most promising recent direction lies in *hybrid systems* that fuse interpretable biomarkers with learned representations, combining the transparency clinicians and practitioners trust with the adaptability that advanced AI enables. For clinicians and practitioners, this means Voice AI tools that can justify their outputs; for engineers and developers, it defines a design space where performance, data efficiency, interpretability, reliability and safety converge.

Foundation models are large-scale, general-purpose machine learning models, typically based on deep learning architectures, that are pre-trained on vast and heterogeneous data and can be adapted, often termed as fine-tuning, toward a broader range of desired tasks. They serve as the 'foundation' for various applications across different domains. Examples include GPT [4], BERT [5], and LLaMA [6], all of which are built on transformer architectures and have been used for applications in natural language processing (NLP), image recognition, and multimodal learning. In healthcare, foundation models are beginning to influence specialized areas such as speech and voice disorders. Yet whether speech-based foundation models can extend to voice, which reflects not only linguistic but also physiological and emotional information, remains an open question.

To develop a *domain-specific* voice foundation model, the model should be trained on large, diverse datasets of vocal recordings, and later fine-tuned on clinically annotated datasets, whereby the model ideally learns to recognize patterns that might indicate the presence of disorders, such as hoarseness or tremors in the voice. However, such data are far scarcer and more ethically sensitive than the web-scale corpora used for speech, raising challenges of privacy, bias, and representativeness [7]. Despite these constraints, the principle of large-scale pre-training remains promising. Foundation models, particularly those trained for spoken communication, can be fine-tuned to identify voice disorders, track patient progress during treatment, and even provide diagnostic support to clinicians.

6.1.2 Trade-off Between Model Groups

While the previous section outlined the range of modeling strategies used in Voice AI, understanding how these models differ in practice requires examining the trade-offs that drive their design and adoption. Each approach, statistical, classical machine learning, deep learning, or foundation-based, occupies a distinct position along a continuum of data dependence, interpretability, and scalability. Recognizing these contrasts is crucial for matching a model to the constraints of real-world clinical use and to the practitioners world. Choosing the right modeling approach for Voice AI is less about algorithmic sophistication and more about balancing practical constraints: data availability, interpretability, and clinical reliability. Feature-based machine-learning models embed domain expertise and are easier to validate, but they scale poorly and capture limited acoustic complexity. Deep-learning models, by contrast, can extract nuanced temporal and spectral cues directly from raw signals, yet their reliance on large, diverse datasets makes them difficult to train and generalize in clinical settings where data are scarce or heterogeneous. These trade-offs are not purely technical, they shape how Voice AI tools are perceived and trusted in practice. Clinicians often favor interpretable, stable models, while engineers push for higher accuracy through scale and automation. The emerging middle ground lies in hybrid approaches and foundation models, which combine learned representations with domain-aware fine-tuning. Understanding and explicitly managing these trade-offs is essential for building voice AI systems that are not only high-performing but also deployable, safe and trustworthy. The following section examines these contextual factors, data, infrastructure, and trust, that ultimately determine which modeling approach is viable for deployment in real-world Voice AI applications.

6.2 Factors Affecting Modelling Choices in Voice AI

Developing AI models for voice disorders involves multiple interdependent factors that influence both their design and their clinical usability. These factors not only directly impact the feasibility of developing the voice models but also their acceptability and trustworthiness, ultimately determining whether they can be successfully deployed in clinical practice [8]. The context of the application, in other words, the deployment scenario in which the model will be used, the targeted user group, and the intended clinical function is critical, especially within the evolving landscape of global AI regulation [9]. For example, a model to automatically predict the GRBAS score from a voice input when applied in a clinical setting [1, 10, 11] must demonstrate high output accuracy and reliability, and the ability to generalize to unseen patients and cohorts [12]. Equally important, clinical users must be able to understand the model's reasoning to the decision; transparent and interpretable decision-making is central to establishing trust. This requires that the model can 'explain' its decisions to the users [13]. The factors shaping these outcomes can be grouped into *four broad categories*, as illustrated in Fig. 6.3: dataset, features, metrics of evaluation, and reproducibility of the reported results. The sections that follow discuss each in turn. While this list is not exhaustive, it highlights the

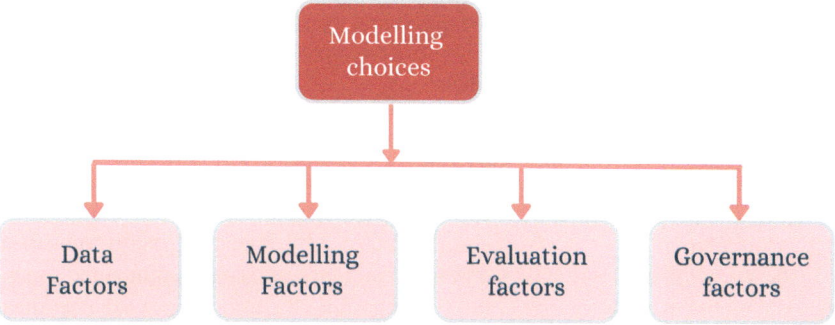

Fig. 6.3 Illustration of the factors that influence the design choices while developing voice AI models

considerations most relevant to the design and deployment of Voice AI systems for the clinician and practitioner's world.

6.2.1 Dataset Factors

Dataset characteristics are the most influential factor determining Voice AI model design, performance, and generalizability. As demonstrated in Fig. 6.4, these can be organized into four interrelated dimensions: type and source, size and data splitting, sample (population) structure, and demographics.

1. *Quality of voice dataset*: Noise and distortions in the voice data can impair not only the training of a voice model but also its deployment, for instance, its clinical use or telehealth integration. If the quality of the training data does not match the quality of the deployment data, a phenomenon known as distribution shift [14], model performance can degrade unpredictably, and the output of the model may deviate from expected outcomes. However, it is non-trivial to control the

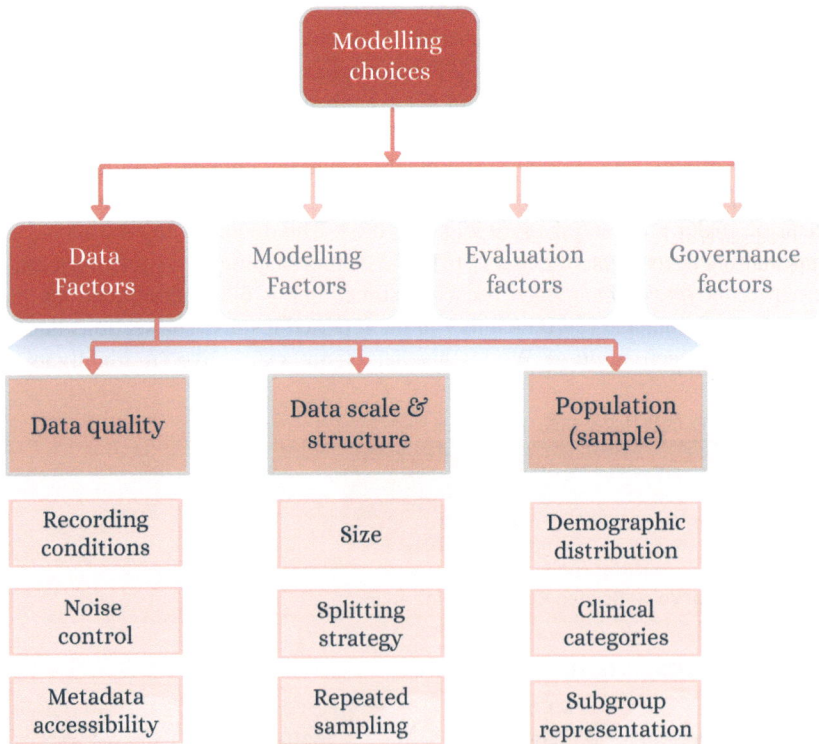

Fig. 6.4 Flow diagram depicting the sub-factors under the dataset design that influence model choices

voice data quality, as the sources of noise in voice data can be from multiple sources that may not be accounted for, for example, inconsistent hardware, microphone quality, acoustic-recording environments, distance of voice source from the microphone, etc. [15]. There is a lack of standardized protocols and metadata conventions for voice-data management; the earliest consensus on it was released only recently [16]. Future clinical and research datasets should therefore emphasize consistent recording procedures, transparent documentation of device and environment metadata, and systematic quality-control checks for noise and artifacts. These practices would support reproducible and clinically reliable Voice AI development.

2. *Dataset scale, availability, and accessibility*: The amount of available and usable data strongly influences the choice between classical machine learning and deep-learning models. Dataset size is commonly quantified in terms of the number of voice samples and the available labels (e.g. 'healthy' or 'disease X') for each sample. Large datasets allow for the use of complex and data-intensive deep-learning models, which can learn intricate patterns within the voice signals from the data. In contrast, smaller datasets may require more traditional machine learning models like SVMs, decision trees, or even linear models, which are less prone to overfitting with limited data. In voice applications where data scarcity remains a barrier, techniques such as transfer learning, data augmentation and federated learning may be employed to enhance model performance. Within clinical and healthcare applications, limited dataset size and restricted data sharing are recurring constrains, often due to the regulations around *private* and *ethical* handling of sensitive healthcare data [17]. Future clinical datasets should therefore prioritize mechanisms for secure data federation, standardized annotation protocols, and transparent documentation of data-splitting strategies to ensure comparability and reproducibility across sites. Establishing shared benchmark datasets and reporting templates would further strengthen evidence accumulation in Voice AI research. While dataset scale constrains model complexity, population structure determines whether the learned relationships hold across diverse speakers, a challenge discussed below.

3. *Population structure and demographics*: Another quality aspect is the diversity of the subjects and the representation in the dataset. Population (sample) diversity, across age, gender, linguistic background, and health status, is a critical determinant of a model's fairness and external validity. Data samples over a broad age range, genders, and health status (controls, vocal cancer, voice co-morbidities) allow developers to identify the operational boundaries of Voice AI models and evaluate whether they generalize across subgroups. For instance, before deploying an automated GRBAS assessment tool in the clinic [1], it is essential to identify which age groups the model performs the best for and if it performs equally well for all genders and shows consistent outcomes toward the expected user groups [9]. Equally important is the dataset's internal structure. Repeated samples from the same individual, if not accounted for during training or cross-validation, can lead to information leakage and artificially inflated accuracy estimates [18]. To prevent this, future dataset protocols should document

subject identifiers, control for within-speaker correlations, and adopt subject-level data splits for model evaluation. Beyond demographic balance, transparent reporting of population composition and subgroup-level results should become standard practice in Voice AI research. Such reporting would support reproducibility, facilitate cross-study comparison, and promote equitable model deployment across diverse clinical populations.Population design completes the data-centric foundation of Voice AI. The next step is to evaluate how these datasets interact with model objectives, metrics, and computational constraints, a topic addressed in the following section.

6.2.2 Evaluation Factors

Designing the evaluation of Voice AI models is as critical as designing the models themselves. This step determines whether model performance reflects true generalization or merely the ability to fit a specific dataset. The sub-factors influencing evaluation design are summarized in Fig. 6.5. Together, these elements also contribute to the general reliability and reproducibility of any Voice AI study and goes a

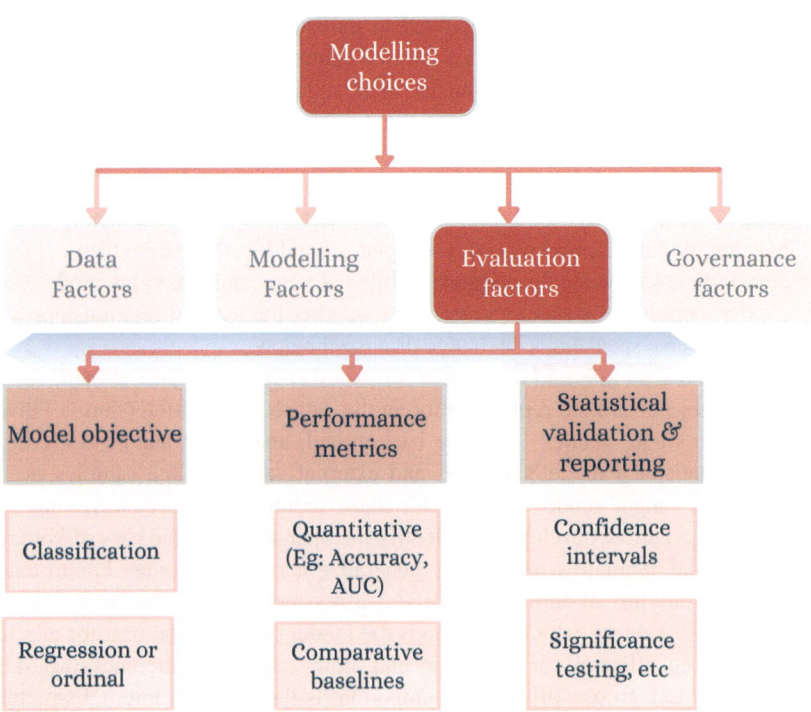

Fig. 6.5 Flow diagram depicting the sub-dimensions under the evaluation factors, that influence model choices

step further towards deployment. Note that the optimum design of experiments for testing AI is not yet standardized, but there is a growing discourse around it with regulations and reporting guidelines [9, 19, 20].

1. *Model Objective*: The desired goal of the model dictates the objective or loss function that should be used in the model. For instance, when an SVM is used for the classification of Parkinson's disorder based on voice input, the loss function tries to maximize the margin between the voice samples and the binary decision boundary [2]. In contrast, when automatically predicting the GRBAS score, which can be seen as continuous or ordinal outcomes [1, 10], the regression loss function during training would minimize the mean squared error (MSE) or the mean absolute error (MAE). Clearly specifying the objective, classification or regression, is essential for choosing valid evaluation metrics and avoiding misinterpretation of results.
2. *Performance Metrics*: The metrics used to test and evaluate AI models rely on the model objectives and the outcomes. For a binary classification outcome, e.g. 'healthy' and 'disease X,' accuracy, specificity, and sensitivity are commonly used. The area under the receiver operating characteristics curve (AUC-ROC) quantifies the performance across decision thresholds. For continuous regression, the MSE or the MAE is most commonly used. Correlation coefficients or ordinal-aware metrics can complement them when clinical grading is involved. Model evaluation should not rely on a single metric. Most metrics, when employed in isolation, provide only a 'snapshot' of the model performance, and can be misleading [18]. Future studies should therefore report a panel of complementary metrics, including precision-recall trade-offs and calibration measures, to ensure fair assessment across cohorts.
3. *Real-Time Processing and Computational Costs*: [3, 21] Statistical Validation: Beyond point estimates of performance, statistical rigor is essential to establish confidence in the results. Reported metrics should include confidence intervals or p-values and, where multiple hypotheses are tested, appropriate correction for multiple comparisons. Pre-registered analysis plans and transparent reporting of evaluation procedures will further strengthen credibility and replicability [18].

6.2.3 Governance Factors

Acceptability of an AI model in high-stakes application scenarios like healthcare and clinical contexts [9, 17] is strongly influenced by the amount of trust the domain experts (clinicians and medical doctors) have in the model. This trust is often tempered by how much the experts are able to interpret the decisions yielded by the AI model (e.g. 'input voice sample has Parkinson's disease with X certainty'). Furthermore, the reproducibility and consistency of the scientific results and model outcomes for different target groups also impact this trust (Fig. 6.6).

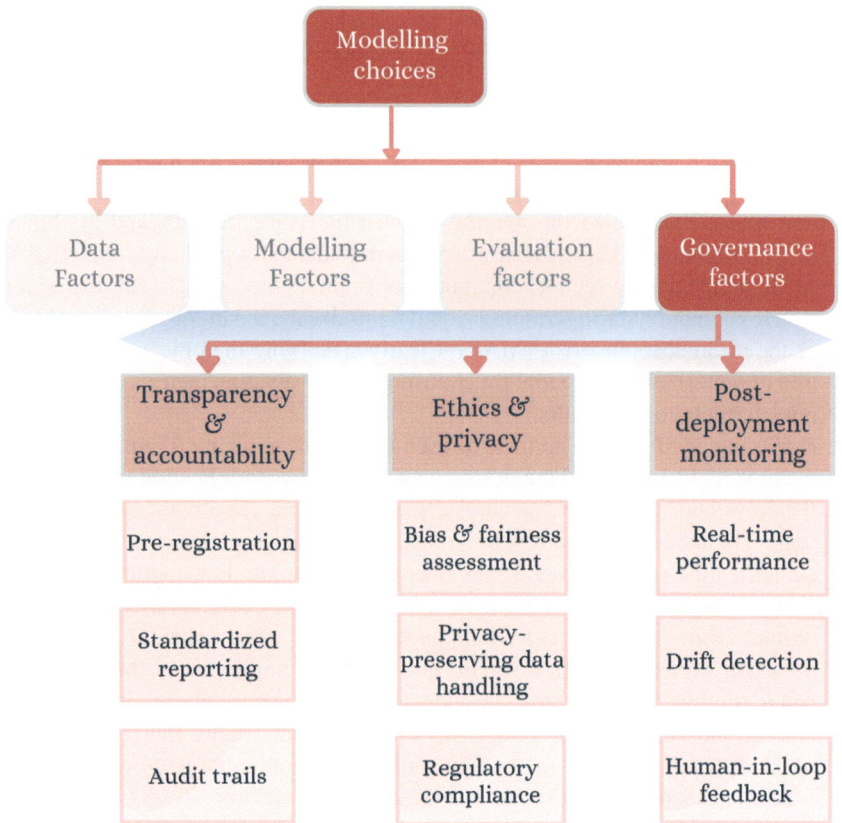

Fig. 6.6 Flow diagram depicting the sub-elements of governance factors

1. *Interpretability and explainability*: While the more complex deep-learning models can offer excellent performance, they are often criticized for being 'black-box' models, offering little interpretability. For clinicians diagnosing and treating voice disorders, the ability to interpret model outputs, i.e., understanding which vocal features contribute to a diagnosis, is often just as important as accuracy. In such cases, models like decision trees or logistic regression may be preferable due to their transparency, even if they sacrifice some accuracy. Although methods that enable explainability and interpretability in deep-learning models exist, the domain is an active research field [22]. Future deployments should prioritize explainable-by-design architectures and integrate visualization tools that make model reasoning accessible to non-technical users. Explainability and interpretability of models are highly encouraged also within the scope of AI regulation [13]. Hence, it is necessary to include domain experts and end-users in the discussion on model type (classical machine-learning or deep learning) choices.

2. *Ethical and privacy considerations*: The uniqueness of voice data is that while its production is founded in a biological-physiological process, it is also a social signal. Therefore, voice data can reflect not just the physique but also a social identity in the form of demographic characteristics like age, gender, or accent. While developing AI models for voice disorders, it is therefore essential to reflect on the modelling choices that might introduce bias [23] and choose models that either minimize bias or allow for adjustments [24]. Ethical considerations also extend to patient privacy, particularly if models require extensive amounts of personal data [17]. Before deployment, during model test and evaluation, it is necessary to establish that the model is legally and ethically sound while still delivering performance.
3. *Pre-registration*: There is a well-established procedure to collect evidence in clinical and medical science on the effectiveness of a certain treatment or intervention [25]. If AI models are introduced in the medical pipeline, either as a primary tool or as a tool aiding doctors, they should be placed at the same level for evaluation. Pre-registering AI studies in healthcare can not only be an aid in ensuring consistency and reliability [12] of AI models but also address the reproducibility crises of AI in healthcare [18].
4. *Real-Time Processing and Computational Costs*: Depending on whether the application requires real-time voice analysis, model complexity and processing power must be considered. Real-time processing places constraints on latency, memory, and computational resources. In these cases, models that prioritize speed over absolute accuracy, such as smaller neural networks or traditional machine learning algorithms, might be more suitable. The computational power available for training and deploying models directly impacts model choice. Deep learning models typically require GPUs or specialized hardware for training and inference, whereas traditional machine learning models can be deployed on more standard hardware. Deployment scenarios (e.g. hospital or clinic), budgetary constraints, and available resources can therefore influence whether a high-performing, resource-intensive model is feasible for the clinical-voice application [21].

6.3 Summary

Selecting the optimal AI model for voice biomarker analysis is a multidimensional. process that extends beyond technical performance. It requires balancing data quality, modeling complexity, evaluation rigor, and governance oversight to ensure the that voice AI systems are accurate, interpretable, and clinically deployable. The framework presented in this chapter links four pillars from biomarker-informed data to post-deployment monitoring, emphasizing reproducibility and trust as continuous obligations. Meaningful progress in voice AI depends on close collaboration among clinicians, engineers, and ethicists throughout the model lifecycle. Ultimately, responsible voice AI is not a static pipeline but a governed learning system that evolves with clinical practice.

References

1. Kojima T, Fujimura S, Hasebe K, Okanoue Y, Shuya O, Yuki R, Shoji K, Hori R, Kishimoto Y, Omori K. Objective assessment of pathological voice using artificial intelligence based on the GRBAS scale. J Voice. 2024;38(3):561–6. https://doi.org/10.1016/j.jvoice.2021.11.021.
2. Costantini G, Cesarini V, Di Leo P, Amato F, Suppa A, Asci F, et al. Artificial intelligence-based voice assessment of patients with Parkinson's disease off and on treatment: machine vs. deep-learning comparison. Sensors (Basel). 2023;23(4):2293. https://doi.org/10.3390/s23042293.
3. Clemmensen LKH, Lønfeldt NN, Das S, Lund NL, Uhre VF, Mora-Jensen AC, Pretzmann L, Uhre CF, Ritter M, Korsbjerg NLJ, Hagstrøm J, Thoustrup CL, Clemmesen IT, Plessen KJ, Pagsberg AK. Associations Between the Severity of Obsessive-Compulsive Disorder and Vocal Features in Children and Adolescents: Protocol for a Statistical and Machine Learning Analysis. JMIR Res Protoc. 2022 Oct 28;11(10):e39613. https://doi.org/10.2196/39613.
4. Achiam J, Adler S, Agarwal S, Ahmad L, Akkaya I, Aleman FL, Almeida D, Altenschmidt J, Altman S, Anadkat S, Avila R. Gpt-4 technical report. arXiv:2303.08774v6 [cs.CL]. 2024.
5. Kenton JD, Toutanova LK. Bert: Pre-training of deep bidirectional transformers for language understanding. In Proceedings of naacL-HLT 2019 Jun 2. (Vol. 1, p. 2).
6. Touvron H, Lavril T, Izacard G, Martinet X, Lachaux MA, Lacroix T, Rozière B, Goyal N, Hambro E, Azhar F, Rodriguez A. Llama: Open and efficient foundation language models. arXiv:2302.13971. 2023 Feb 27.
7. Bommasani, R. (2021). On the opportunities and risks of foundation models. arXiv preprint arXiv:2108.07258.
8. Giddings R, Joseph A, Callender T, Janes SM, van der Schaar M, Sheringham J, Navani N. Factors influencing clinician and patient interaction with machine learning-based risk prediction models: a systematic review. Lancet Digit Health. 2024;6(2):e131–44. https://doi.org/10.1016/S2589-7500(23)00241-8.
9. Corrêa NK, Mönig JM. Catalog of general ethical requirements for AI certification. arXiv:2408.12289. 2024 Aug 22.
10. Hidaka S, Lee Y, Nakanishi M, Wakamiya K, Nakagawa T, Kaburagi T. Automatic GRBAS scoring of pathological voices using deep learning and a small set of labeled voice data. J Voice. 2022; https://doi.org/10.1016/j.jvoice.2022.10.020.
11. Yamamoto N, Onoda K. Item-specific analysis of hoarseness to detect aspiration after cardiac surgery: an exploratory study of adopting an iPhone application "GRBASZero". Indian J Thorac Cardiovasc Surg. 2024 Nov;40(6):684–9. https://doi.org/10.1007/s12055-024-01758-x.
12. Liu Y, Zhang C, Liu Z, Li J. Reliability and validity of GRBASzero in clinical environments. J Voice. 2024 Jul 9;S0892-1997(24):00199–1. https://doi.org/10.1016/j.jvoice.2024.06.018.
13. Panigutti C, Hamon R, Hupont I, Llorca DF, Yela DF, Junklewitz H, et al. The role of explainable AI in the context of the AI Act. 2022 ACM conference on fairness, accountability, and transparency. 2023:1139–50. https://doi.org/10.1145/3593013.3594069.
14. Quiñonero-Candela J, Sugiyama M, Schwaighofer A, Lawrence ND, editors. Dataset shift in machine learning. MIT Press; 2022 Jun 7.
15. Evangelista E, Kale R, McCutcheon D, Rameau A, Gelbard A, Powell M, et al. Current practices in voice data collection and limitations to voice AI research: a National Survey. Laryngoscope. 2024 Mar;134(3):1333–9. https://doi.org/10.1002/lary.31052.
16. Lechien JR, Geneid A, Bohlender JE, Cantarella G, Avellaneda JC, Desuter G, et al. Consensus for voice quality assessment in clinical practice: guidelines of the European laryngological society and Union of the European Phoniatricians. Eur Arch Otorrinolaringol. 2023 Dec;280(12):5459–73. https://doi.org/10.1007/s00405-023-08211-6.
17. Voigt P, Von dem Bussche A. The eu general data protection regulation (gdpr). A practical guide. 1st ed. Cham: Springer; 2017.;10(3152676). p. 10–5555.
18. Varoquaux G, Cheplygina V. Machine learning for medical imaging: methodological failures and recommendations for the future. NPJ Digit Med. 2022;5(1):48. https://doi.org/10.1038/s41746-022-00592-y.

19. Vasey B, Nagendran M, Campbell B, Clifton DA, Collins GS, Denaxas S, et al. Reporting guideline for the early-stage clinical evaluation of decision support systems driven by artificial intelligence: DECIDE-AI. Nat Med. 2022 May;28(5):924–33. https://doi.org/10.1038/s41591-022-01772-9.
20. Liu X, Cruz Rivera S, Moher D, Calvert MJ, Denniston AK. Reporting guidelines for clinical trial reports for interventions involving artificial intelligence: the CONSORT-AI extension. Lancet Digit Health. 2020 Oct;2(10):e537–48. https://doi.org/10.1016/S2589-7500(20)30218-1.
21. Souter NE, Racey C, Bhagwat N, Wilkinson R, Duncan NW, Samuel G, Lannelongue L, Selvan R, Rae CL. Comparing the carbon footprint of fMRI data processing and analysis approaches. Imaging Neurosci (Camb). 2025 Jun 16;3:IMAG.a.36.
22. Samek W, Montavon G, Vedaldi A, Hansen LK, Müller KR. Explainable AI: interpreting, explaining and visualizing deep learning. Springer Nature; 2019. https://doi.org/10.1007/978-3-030-28954-6.
23. Wiens J, Saria S, Sendak M, Ghassemi M, Liu VX, Doshi-Velez F, Jung K, Heller K, Kale D, Saeed M, Ossorio PN, Thadaney-Israni S, Goldenberg A. Do no harm: a roadmap for responsible machine learning for health care. Nat Med. 2019;25(9):1337–40. https://doi.org/10.1038/s41591-019-0548-6.
24. Zicari RV, Brusseau J, Blomberg SN, Christensen HC, Coffee M, Ganapini MB, et al. On assessing trustworthy AI in healthcare. Machine learning as a supportive tool to recognize cardiac arrest in emergency calls. Front Hum Dyn [Internet]. 2021;3 https://doi.org/10.3389/fhumd.2021.673104.
25. Drazen JM, Haug CJ. Trials of AI interventions must be preregistered. NEJM AI. 2024;1(4) https://doi.org/10.1056/aie2400146.

Open Access This chapter is licensed under the terms of the Creative Commons Attribution-NonCommercial-NoDerivatives 4.0 International License (http://creativecommons.org/licenses/by-nc-nd/4.0/), which permits any noncommercial use, sharing, distribution and reproduction in any medium or format, as long as you give appropriate credit to the original author(s) and the source, provide a link to the Creative Commons license and indicate if you modified the licensed material. You do not have permission under this license to share adapted material derived from this chapter or parts of it.

The images or other third party material in this chapter are included in the chapter's Creative Commons license, unless indicated otherwise in a credit line to the material. If material is not included in the chapter's Creative Commons license and your intended use is not permitted by statutory regulation or exceeds the permitted use, you will need to obtain permission directly from the copyright holder.

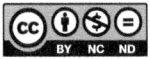

Voice-Related Biomarkers

Mieke Moerman and Mette Pedersen

7.1 Introduction

The Voice-related Biomarkers Committee of the Union of European Phoniatricians (UEP) was established in May 2023, with the aim of exploring possible biomarkers in phoniatrics and starting research into voice-related biomarkers, referring to a consensus paper together with the European Laryngology Society [1]. In 1998, the National Institutes of Health Biomarkers Definitions Working Group defined a biomarker as "a characteristic that is objectively measured and evaluated as an indicator of normal biological processes, pathogenic processes, or pharmacologic responses to a therapeutic intervention." This means that molecular, histologic, radiographic, or physiologic measures are types of biomarkers. A biomarker must have a prognostic/predictive value and a monetary value [2].

Presentation from the commission on voice-related biomarkers at the second Joint Meeting of the Union of European Phoniatrics (UEP)/European Academy of Phoniatrics (EAP) with the British Laryngology Association (BLA).

M. Moerman
Board Member UEP/EAP, TelePHON.digital BV, Founder UEP Biomarkers Committee, St Martens Latem, Belgium

M. Pedersen (✉)
The Medical Center, Copenhagen, Denmark
e-mail: M.f.pedersen@dadlnet.dk

7.1.1 Definition

By definition, a biomarker fulfills certain conditions and at least the following three:

Specificity. This means that the objectively measured characteristic does what it claims it does. A narrow focus is essential for good specificity.
Effectiveness. A biomarker has to make sense. From a clinical-practical standpoint, a good biomarker can help prevent death or life-threatening situations.
Efficiency. In view of social costs, a biomarker must be efficient, and the process for determining a biomarker must be cost-effective in terms of both the technical aspect and the time spent. So the simpler the process, the better. The more accessible, the better.

Narrowing down to the topic of "voice-related biomarkers," more specifically, the UEP voice-related biomarkers committee examined the literature to see what already existed—what is already known as an innovative subject.

It appears that the term "voice as a digital biomarker" occurs frequently, especially in Parkinson's disease, often based on free speech but also on vowels, based on telephone recordings, and with the use of machine learning (ML) [3–33].

Although it appears trivial, the content and subjects of phoniatrics and, more specifically, what voice means to a phoniatrician, have to be described. Phoniatrics distinguishes between sound production, which takes place at the level of vocal folds, and the audible end result, speech, where the sound produced undergoes abundant influences, such as resonator and articulatory influences during its passage through the vocal tract. In phoniatrics, there is also a distinction between speech and language. The latter requires accurate cognitive functioning, e.g., word finding, rhythm, and prosody.

7.1.2 Glottal Function

The three most important and highly relevant functions of the glottis are to facilitate ventilation, facilitate phonation, and provide airway protection. In phoniatrics, "voice-related biomarkers" are characteristics of the three aforementioned glottal functions. At the same time, it is necessary to be able to evaluate and objectively measure these characteristics. To make the biomarker as effective and efficient as possible, the challenge lies in matching it with life-threatening situations on the one hand and with simple and clear processes on the other. Therefore, the UEP biomarker voice committee approaches the physiological events of the glottis, more specifically, the glottal closure. The glottal closure bridges the gap between sound production and swallowing. The closure of the vocal cords is paramount for both physiological processes and affects a huge number of people.

7.1.3 Prevalence of Swallowing and Voice Problems

It appears that swallowing problems occur in 4% of our adult population and dysphonia in 3–9%. Furthermore, it is an important aspect that dysphagia and dysphonia

Table 7.1 Frequency of dysphagia and dysphonia. Frequency of Parkinson's disease in connection with other disorders

Individuals:	
1 dysphagia: 4% of the adult population	
2 dysphonia: 3–9% of the adult population	
Patients:	
3 Parkinson's disease: 80%	
4 Alzheimer's disease: 84–93%	
5 head and neck oncology: +/− 40%	

today have a prevalence of up to 80% in Parkinson's disease, up to 84–93% in Alzheimer's, and 40% in head and neck oncology patients, as shown in Table 7.1. Parkinson's disease is the second most frequent neurodegenerative disorder.

7.1.4 Voice-Related Biomarkers

In the literature, a variety of diseases are associated with voice changes as a symptom and vice versa: voice changes can indicate illness or the onset of disease. Among neurodegenerative diseases, e.g., in Parkinson's disease, up to 80% of early-stage Parkinson's patients have voice problems. We have dived deeply into the literature for the last 10 years (2013–2023) and studied 47 papers published between 2013 and 2019, mainly without artificial intelligence (AI), and 51 papers published between 2019 and 2023, including 20 papers based on AI. In Table 7.2, validation is shown based on 7561 patients (23 papers without numbers) and 1513 controls. Most studies are on early and moderate cases of Parkinson's disease. Seven papers present the results of deep brain treatment. Mostly, validation in non-AI papers is HNR, F0, intensity, jitter, shimmer, and VHI. Also, in non-AI papers, SNR, MPT, spectrography, and LTAS, cepstrum analysis, VRP, and GRBAS are used. Praat is used in both non-AI and some AI cases. AI is used for validation in 24 papers during 2013–2023, and is often based on many more parameters. The meaning of the abbreviations can be found in Chap. 2.

It appears that the most frequently used voice-related parameters for evaluating Parkinson's disease are acoustical features and the Voice Handicap Index (VHI). The perceptual evaluation (GRBAS test) and airflow with MPT are also used. Laryngoscopy is less commonly applied. The multidimensionality of voice is emphasized, which will be discussed in the next section. To conclude the literature review, there are problems because many reports concerning voice-related biomarkers in Alzheimer's, multiple sclerosis, rheumatoid arthritis, mental health (depression, schizophrenia), cardiovascular disease, diabetes, COVID, respiratory conditions, etc., conflate voice with speech and language: articulation, rhythm, semantics, word finding, etc.

The manuscripts in this book are not entirely coherent with our phoniatric definition of voice physiological processes, production, or voice changes. But voice is not the same as speech. Voice must be viewed separately from the influences of speech and language. After all, pure voice production concerns events at the level of the vocal folds and has nothing to do with resonance, articulation, or prosody. Pure voice production is complicated enough alone. Focusing on mere voice production, multidimensionality must be taken into account.

Table 7.2 Non-AI papers. The table shows the non-AI voice analysis in the papers; it is noted that fundamental frequency is mostly used, as well as jitter, shimmer, HNR, and others. It is noted that in the overview of articles, 24 include AI, and they are later discussed. Copyright: Pedersen M (2025) [34], redistributed under the terms of the Creative Commons Attribution License (CC BY 4.0)

Parameters.	Total
No. of patients (cases)	7561 (23 without no.)
Prospective articles	25
Randomized articles	5
Retrospective articles	6
Controls	1513
HNR	**23**
SNR	8
F0 (+ SD)	**40**
Intensity	**24**
Jitter ABS/%	**29**
Shimmer ABS/%	**23**
Spektral and LTAS	9
Cepstrum analysis	5
VRP	4
VHI	**25**
MPT	14
GRBAS	10
Deep brain surgery	7
Telephone calls	3
Praat reference	13
AI	**24**
Deep learning	9
Laryngoscopy	6

7.1.5 Multidimensionality

Acoustics alone is not sufficient. But linguistics, semantics, and vocabulary do not reflect glottal function. Relying on the publication of Lechien et al. [1], a good understanding of voice physiology is based on five dimensions, as seen in Fig. 7.1: self-assessment, perception, visualization, acoustics, and aerodynamics, as symbolized.

This implies that acoustics alone is not sufficient to obtain clear and accurate voice-related biomarkers reflecting voice production. We should embrace more dimensions, keeping in mind that the administration process is as simple as possible for the individual. Until today, the intervention of a healthcare provider is required as far as the 'visualization' dimension is concerned, and also as far as the perceptual assessment is concerned. Except for acoustics and some of the aerodynamic measurements, none of these dimensions can be objectively measured. Scores of evaluations are made for patient complaints and listener evaluation, usable with AI.

This brings us to future perspectives on innovation: to get a digital test that the person could perform and that could be used for screening, triage, diagnosis, therapeutic monitoring, and self-monitoring. The AI foundation software gives this possibility for the future.

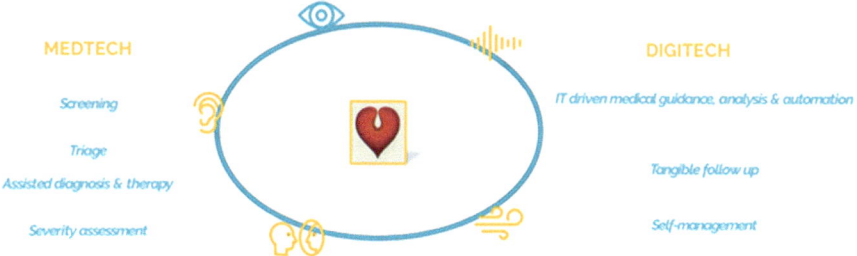

Fig. 7.1 Personalized guidance—Virtual testing. Available/Affordable/Accessible

7.1.6 Preliminary Clinical Protocol

This protocol includes easily accessible parameters with the potential to lead to a multidimensional biomarker for glottal closure function. We suggest keeping at least the following parameters, considering their importance in the glottal closure function:

- Self-assessment
- Perception
- Acoustics
- Visualization
- Aerodynamics

The committee suggests keeping at least the following parameters, considering their importance in the glottal closure function:

- GRBAS test.
- VHI (related to glottal closure function/voicing.)
- HNR, (NHR, and voicing quantification parameters.)
- Visualization (with Laryngoscopy, Stroboscopy, and High-Speed Films.)
- MPT, (Glottal Closure Quotient, inverse filtering.)

(For full names of the abbreviations, see Chap. 2).

7.2 Conclusion

Voice is different from speech and language; voice is multi-dimensional. The glottal closure function is vitally important. Determining a voice-related biomarker should be simple and straightforward, affordable, largely accessible, and available. Presumably, AI is needed to determine the weight of the different dimensions to obtain a multidimensional, accurate biomarker.

The committee decided to work on defining biomarkers that reveal glottal function. As the three most important and relevant functions of the glottis are to facilitate ventilation, to provide phonation, and to protect the airways, the focus primarily lies on the glottal closure. Good glottal closure is not only necessary for a good voice but also to prevent aspiration. The AI foundation software gives the possibility of a well-defined voice-related biomarker in the future.

References

1. Lechien JR, Geneid A, Bohlender JE, Cantarella G, Avellaneda JC, Desuter G, et al. Consensus for voice quality assessment in clinical practice: guidelines of the European laryngological society and Union of the European Phoniatricians. Eur Arch Otorrinolaringol. 2023;280(12):5459–73. https://doi.org/10.1007/s00405-023-08211-6.
2. Strimbu K, Tavel JA. What are biomarkers? Curr Opin HIV AIDS. 2010;5(6):463–6. https://doi.org/10.1097/COH.0b013e32833ed177.
3. Idrisoglu A, Dallora AL, Anderberg P, Berglund JS. Applied machine learning techniques to diagnose voice-affecting conditions and disorders: systematic literature review. J Med Internet Res. 2023;25:e46105. https://doi.org/10.2196/46105.
4. Worasawate D, Asawaponwiput W, Yoshimura N, Intarapanich A, Surangsrirat D. Classification of Parkinson's disease from smartphone recording data using time-frequency analysis and convolutional neural network. Technol Health Care. 2023;31(2):705–18. https://doi.org/10.3233/THC-220386.
5. Alghamdi NS, Zakariah M, Hoang VT, Elahi MM. Neurogenerative disease diagnosis in Cepstral domain using MFCC with deep learning. Comput Math Methods Med. 2022;2022:4364186. https://doi.org/10.1155/2022/4364186. Retraction in: Comput Math Methods Med 2023 Dec 13;2023:9786412. https://doi.org/10.1155/2023/9786412
6. Ngo QC, Motin MA, Pah ND, Drotár P, Kempster P, Kumar D. Computerized analysis of speech and voice for Parkinson's disease: a systematic review. Comput Methods Prog Biomed. 2022 Nov;226:107133. https://doi.org/10.1016/j.cmpb.2022.107133.
7. Ma J, Zhang Y, Li Y, Zhou L, Qin L, Zeng Y, et al. Deep dual-side learning ensemble model for Parkinson speech recognition. Biomed Signal Process Control. 2021;69:102849. https://doi.org/10.1016/j.bspc.2021.102849.
8. Sahandi Far M, Eickhoff SB, Goni M, Dukart J. Exploring test-retest reliability and longitudinal stability of digital biomarkers for Parkinson disease in the m-power data set: cohort study. J Med Internet Res. 2021;23(9):e26608. https://doi.org/10.2196/26608.
9. Jeancolas L, Petrovska-Delacrétaz D, Mangone G, Benkelfat BE, Corvol JC, Vidailhet M, et al. X-vectors: new quantitative biomarkers for early Parkinson's disease detection from speech. Front Neuroinform. 2021;15:578369. https://doi.org/10.3389/fninf.2021.578369.
10. Gupta S, Patil AT, Purohit M, Parmar M, Patel M, Patil HA, Guido RC. Residual neural network precisely quantifies dysarthria severity-level based on short-duration speech segments. Neural Netw. 2021;139:105–17. https://doi.org/10.1016/j.neunet.2021.02.008.
11. Arora S, Tsanas A. Assessing Parkinson's disease at scale using telephone-recorded speech: insights from the Parkinson's voice initiative. Diagnostics (Basel). 2021;11(10):1892. https://doi.org/10.3390/diagnostics11101892.
12. Yaman O, Ertam F, Tuncer T. Automated Parkinson's disease recognition based on statistical pooling method using acoustic features. Med Hypotheses. 2020 Feb;135:109483. https://doi.org/10.1016/j.mehy.2019.109483.
13. Solana-Lavalle G, Galán-Hernández JC, Rosas-Romero R. Automatic Parkinson disease detection at early stages as a pre-diagnosis tool by using classifiers and a small set of vocal features. J Appl Biomed. 2020;40(1):505–16. https://doi.org/10.1016/j.bbe.2020.01.003.

14. Sisto R, Viziano A, Stefani A, Moleti A, Cerroni R, Liguori C, Garasto E, Pierantozzi M. Lateralization of cochlear dysfunction as a specific biomarker of Parkinson's disease. Brain Commun. 2020;2(2):fcaa144. https://doi.org/10.1093/braincomms/fcaa144.
15. Tougui I, Jilbab A, Mhamdi JE. Analysis of smartphone recordings in time, frequency, and Cepstral domains to classify Parkinson's disease. Healthc Inform Res. 2020 Oct;26(4):274–83. https://doi.org/10.4258/hir.2020.26.4.274.
16. Tracy JM, Özkanca Y, Atkins DC, Hosseini GR. Investigating voice as a biomarker: deep phenotyping methods for early detection of Parkinson's disease. J Biomed Inform. 2020 Apr;104:103362. https://doi.org/10.1016/j.jbi.2019.103362.
17. Gómez P, Mekyska J, Gómez A, Palacios D, Rodellar V, Álvarez A. Characterization of Parkinson's disease dysarthria in terms of speech articulation kinematics. Biomed Signal Process Control. 2019 May;9(52):312–20. https://doi.org/10.1016/j.bspc.2019.04.029.
18. Upadhya SS, Cheeran AN, Nirmal JH. Thomson multitaper MFCC and PLP voice features for early detection of Parkinson disease. Biomed Signal Process Control. 2018;46:293–301. https://doi.org/10.1016/j.bspc.2018.07.019.
19. Moro-Velazquez L, Gomez-Garcia JA, Godino-Llorente JI, Villalba J, Rusz J, Shattuck-Hufnagel S, et al. A forced gaussians based methodology for the differential evaluation of Parkinson's disease by means of speech processing. Biomed Signal Process Control. 2018;48:205–20. https://doi.org/10.1016/j.bspc.2018.10.020.
20. Ma A, Lau KK, Thyagarajan D. Voice changes in Parkinson's disease: what are they telling us? J Clin Neurosci. 2020 Feb;72:1–7. https://doi.org/10.1016/j.jocn.2019.12.029.
21. Postuma RB. Voice changes in prodromal Parkinson's disease: is a new biomarker within earshot? Sleep Med. 2016 Mar;19:148–9. https://doi.org/10.1016/j.sleep.2015.08.019.
22. Wu K, Zhang D, Lu G, Guo Z. Learning acoustic features to detect Parkinson's disease. Neurocomputing (Amst). 2018 Aug;30(318):102–8. https://doi.org/10.1016/j.neucom.2018.08.036.
23. Montaña D, Campos-Roca Y, Pérez CJ. A Diadochokinesis-based expert system considering articulatory features of plosive consonants for early detection of Parkinson's disease. Comput Methods Prog Biomed. 2018 Feb;154:89–97. https://doi.org/10.1016/j.cmpb.2017.11.010.
24. Singh S, Xu W. Robust detection of Parkinson's disease using harvested smartphone voice data: a telemedicine approach. Telemed J E Health. 2020 Mar;26(3):327–34. https://doi.org/10.1089/tmj.2018.0271.
25. Galaz Z, Mekyska J, Mzourek Z, Smekal Z, Rektorova I, Eliasova I, et al. Prosodic analysis of neutral, stress-modified and rhymed speech in patients with Parkinson's disease. Comput Methods Prog Biomed. 2016 Apr;127:301–17. https://doi.org/10.1016/j.cmpb.2015.12.011.
26. Rektorova I, Mekyska J, Janousova E, Kostalova M, Eliasova I, Mrackova M, et al. Speech prosody impairment predicts cognitive decline in Parkinson's disease. Parkinsonism Relat Disord. 2016 Aug;29:90–5. https://doi.org/10.1016/j.parkreldis.2016.05.018.
27. Harris R, Leenders KL, de Jong BM. Speech dysprosody but no music 'dysprosody' in Parkinson's disease. Brain Lang. 2016 Dec;163:1–9. https://doi.org/10.1016/j.bandl.2016.08.008.
28. Mollaei F, Shiller DM, Baum SR, Gracco VL. Sensorimotor control of vocal pitch and formant frequencies in Parkinson's disease. Brain Res. 2016;1646:269–77. https://doi.org/10.1016/j.brainres.2016.06.013.
29. Bayestehtashk A, Asgari M, Shafran I, McNames J. Fully automated assessment of the severity of Parkinson's disease from speech. Comput Speech Lang. 2015 Jan;29(1):172–85. https://doi.org/10.1016/j.csl.2013.12.001.
30. Péron J, Cekic S, Haegelen C, Sauleau P, Patel S, Drapier D, Vérin M, Grandjean D. Sensory contribution to vocal emotion deficit in Parkinson's disease after subthalamic stimulation. Cortex. 2015 Feb;63:172–83. https://doi.org/10.1016/j.cortex.2014.08.023.
31. Miller DB, O'Callaghan JP. Biomarkers of Parkinson's disease: present and future. Metabolism. 2015 Mar;64(3 Suppl 1):S40–6. https://doi.org/10.1016/j.metabol.2014.10.030.

32. Mekyska J, Janousova E, Gomez-Vilda P, Smekal Z, Rektorova I, Eliasova I, et al. Robust and complex approach of pathological speech signal analysis. Neurocomputing (Amst). 2015 May;21(167):94–111. https://doi.org/10.1016/j.neucom.2015.02.085.
33. Skodda S, Flasskamp A, Schlegel U. Instability of syllable repetition as a marker of disease progression in Parkinson's disease: a longitudinal study. Mov Disord. 2011 Jan;26(1):59–64. https://doi.org/10.1002/mds.23382.
34. Pedersen M. Artificial intelligence for screening voice disorders: aspects of risk factors: research article. Am J Med Clin Res Rev. 2025 Feb;4(2):1–8. https://doi.org/10.58372/2835-6276.1254.

Open Access This chapter is licensed under the terms of the Creative Commons Attribution-NonCommercial-NoDerivatives 4.0 International License (http://creativecommons.org/licenses/by-nc-nd/4.0/), which permits any noncommercial use, sharing, distribution and reproduction in any medium or format, as long as you give appropriate credit to the original author(s) and the source, provide a link to the Creative Commons license and indicate if you modified the licensed material. You do not have permission under this license to share adapted material derived from this chapter or parts of it.

The images or other third party material in this chapter are included in the chapter's Creative Commons license, unless indicated otherwise in a credit line to the material. If material is not included in the chapter's Creative Commons license and your intended use is not permitted by statutory regulation or exceeds the permitted use, you will need to obtain permission directly from the copyright holder.

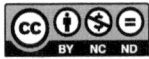

Software and Apps for Glottal Inverse Filtering

8

Ramón Hernández-Villoria

8.1 Introduction

8.1.1 Assessment methods of the glottic space

The glottal space is a small area in the center of the larynx, just 1–3 cm^2, and is of most significant interest in voice assessment. Space closure is the biomechanical basis of the voice's fundamental sound and corresponds to the moment of glottal excitation.

The usual way to observe the glottic level is laryngeal endoscopy (videolaryngostroboscopy), an invasive visual method. The evaluator rates various indicators of glottic function on rating scales. A strobe light allows specific qualitative and quantitative measurements, but it is not all that is needed [1].

Electroglottography is a less invasive method of measuring the opening and closing of the glottal space. It records the variation of electrical potential obtained by placing electrodes superficially on the neck during vocal tasks, generating a wave-shaped trace. Electroglottography cannot resolve the differences in the opening of the anterior part of the glottis in the time domain compared to the posterior part, which is not strictly synchronous [2].

For its part, Glottal inverse filtering (GIF) estimates the source of voiced speech, the glottal volume velocity waveform [3], and has been explained in an earlier chapter. GIF estimates, not measures, the volume velocity waveform, which is an aerodynamic dimension and is the movement caused by a sound wave of a unit volume transmitting through a unit area per unit of time. The function (graphics) and parameterization of this waveform are obtained by software.

R. Hernández-Villoria (✉)
Centro Clínico de Audición y Lenguaje Cealca, Caracas, Venezuela

Hospital de Clínicas Caracas, Caracas, Venezuela

8.1.2 Glottal Inverse Filtering (GIF) Parameters

8.1.2.1 Parameters

They are a compressed numerical form extracted from the estimated function and can be expressed in the time or frequency domains. A parameter in time provides us with how the opening and closing conditions of the glottis change during the emission of the voice. In contrast, a parameter in frequency provides us with information on how glottal excitation affects the harmony of the sound generated. Having this data in numerical form makes identifying events at the glottis level easier.

8.1.2.2 Meaning of Time Domain Parameters

These parameters are time-based quotients [3]. The first one is the *opening quotient* (OQ), or the time the glottis gets open during a period T of voice emission. The *closing quotient* (ClQ) parameter is the result of dividing the closing time by the total cycle time. If the numerical value of the quotient is high, it may mean difficulties in closing. If the value is low, it indicates a short duration and suggests intense and rapid adduction.

Although the *speed quotient's* (SQ) name suggests speed (distance/time), it is a proportion of the open time's duration over the closing time's duration. A high value of the ratio induces the idea of difficulty in closing, while a low value suggests a hyperfunction.

Amplitude domain parameterization methods. The *normalized amplitude quotient* (NAQ) was developed to solve the problem of breathy voices. It is more robust to distortions caused by noise and is based on the amplitude domain rather than directly on time [4].

8.1.2.3 Meaning of Frequency Domain Parameters

Amplitude difference between first and second harmonics (dH1-H2). The increase in the amplitude of the first harmonic is a consequence of the glottal opening [5]. Consequently, if the opening time increases, H1 will increase, causing the difference with H2. For this reason, it is an indicator of a breathy voice and the phonation mode, and is the counterpart of OQ.

The parabolic spectral parameter (PSP) is a numerical value representing the vocal source's spectral decline in terms of its maximum theoretical value. This condition makes it beneficial when audio signals have many different spectral characteristics [6]. If the phonation mode changes in a speech sample, the estimation of OQ and SQ may be less effective than PSP in establishing the influence of glottal opening time on the voice.

Harmonic richness factor (HRF) is "the ratio of the amplitude of the fundamental to the sum of the amplitudes of the harmonics above the fundamental" [7]; therefore, it represents in what proportion the glottal source contributes to the harmony of the entire sound set. *Harmonic to noise ratio* (HNR) estimates the amount of energy that periodic sounds contribute to the aperiodic sounds in the vocal sound [8].

8.1.3 How to Get Waveform and Parameters

GIF has many applications. Essential voice and speech research, voice analysis applications (speaker identification, biometric recognition), speech analysis (emotional contour identification), speech and speech synthesis (voice robots, vocoders, vocal source modeling for text-to-speech), modulation of speech signals (corrections, alterations, simulations, and dissimulations of voice and speech), occupational voice health, singing voice training, in identification of laryngeal pathologies, and also other pathologies different from laryngeal diseases that affect the voice [3, 9–12].

Many acoustic engineering laboratories have developed systems for GIF with different purposes within the range of applications that the method has. As it is difficult to carry out an exhaustive examination of all existing software in this chapter, it has been decided to describe three of them as an example of what can be done with GIF and take into account, above all, the possibility of using them for clinical purposes, that is, the identification of pathologies through voice.

The software packages chosen are Aalto Aparat, Sopran, and Online Lab VCS. The first two are programs for personal computers (PCs) and laptops, while the last is designed for mobile devices (tablets and smartphones).

8.2 Perspectives

8.2.1 Aalto Aparat

Aalto Aparat: The *Aalto Voice Source Analysis and Parameterization Toolkit* is software developed by acoustic engineers and professors of the Department of Signal Processing and Acoustics of the School of Electrical Engineering, Aalto University, Finland, from 2003 to 2008 in the first stage and in 2015 in its second stage. It has had two revisions, and its latest version is v.2.1. It is a package under the GNU LGPL license.

The package is downloaded from the address http://research.spa.aalto.fi/projects/aparat/. [13] Its manual and FAQ are available at http://aalto.fi/aparat. The published reference describing the release of the current version is [13, 14].

Aalto Aparat is PC software based on MATLAB. It is an.exe file and only runs on Microsoft Windows® operating systems. The software works with two different GIF methods: the QCP (quasi-closed phase analysis) method, the default method, and the IAIF (iterative adaptive inverse filtering) method. As explained, QCP offers more quality and fine-tuning results, while IAIF is more robust and preferable when there is a low signal-to-noise ratio (SNR). The software runs optimally with samples from 0.5 to 10 seconds long.

It is a very user-friendly software that quickly delivers its signal analysis. It is necessary to install the program. With version 2.1, there is no need to install any MATLAB components. When you open the program, the main window with the main menus and the signal view window are displayed. It does not directly capture signals. The audio signals must be recorded by other means in .wav format and saved in a directory from which they will be captured by the program using the Open directory action in the file menu. However, the analysis result can be saved as a .mat file or exported as a .wav file.

Figure 8.1 shows the main window and the options in each menu. In the main window, we can select the GIF method (QCP or IAIF) for the analysis and other settings, which already have default values but can be modified (Fig. 8.2). The program supports the possibility of using a second channel for the integral electroglottographic signal in the analysis.

The *Windows* menu allows you to show the parameterization values of the calculated graphic function if the *Show* parameters action is chosen. The parameters delivered are NAQ, AQ, ClQ, OQ, QOQ, SQ (time-based), and dH1-H2, PSP, HNR, and HRF (frequency-based) (Fig. 8.3).

The software allows you to display other windows with graphs calculated from the original GIF: spectra, z-plane, phase-plane, and vocal tract. However, the parameterization results (values) cannot be exported in a summary form in files of the datasheet class.

8.2.2 Sopran

Sopran is a sound processing and analysis .exe package designed by Swedish Associate Professor Svante Granqvist of the KTH Royal Institute of Technology, Fleminsberg, Sweden. It is only executable on Windows OS. The latest version is v. 1.0.28, compiled in November 2023. It was initially designed in 2009. Its copyright belongs to Tolvan Data, a company created by Granqvist. The software is freeware and can be downloaded from https://www.tolvan.com/index.php?page=/sopran/sopran.php [15].

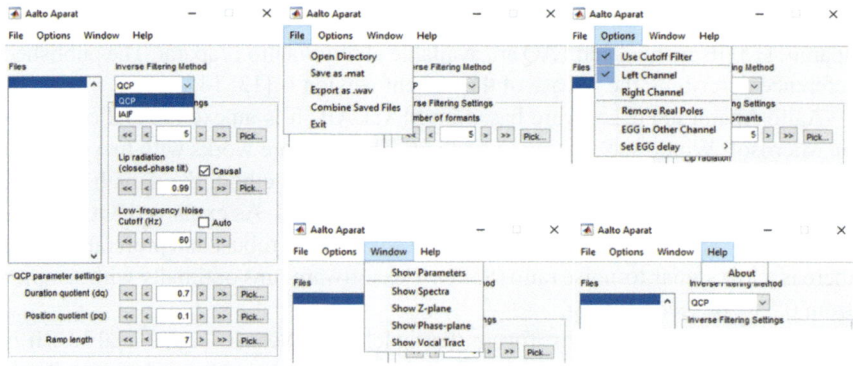

Fig. 8.1 Aalto Aparat. The Aalto Aparat main window and the menus of this window are open. Screenshot of Aalto Aparat. © Paavo Alku et al., Aalto University

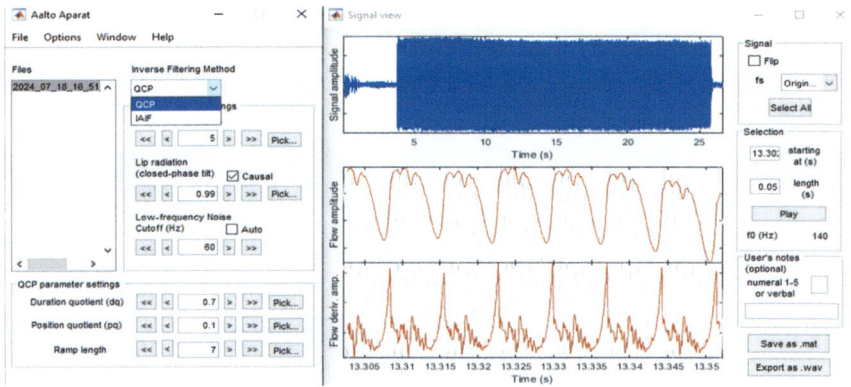

Fig. 8.2 Aalto Aparat. Main window and signal view window. An audio signal.wav file has been opened from a directory. The small box contains a drop-down excerpt of the available GIF analysis methods. By default, QCP is selected. Screenshot of Aalto Aparat. © Paavo Alku et al., Aalto University

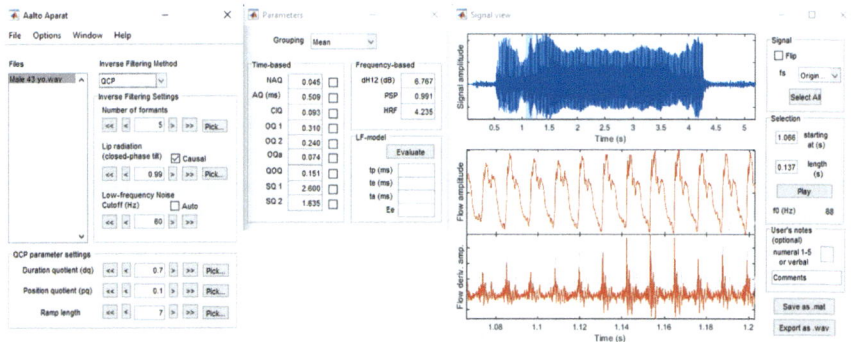

Fig. 8.3 Aalto Aparat with a loaded voice audio signal. Aalto Aparat. Main window, parameterization window, and signal window with a loaded voice audio signal. Screenshot of Aalto Aparat. © Paavo Alku et al., Aalto University

Once downloaded, the program is portable and does not require installation. Its author declares that the software is barely under development and has no documentation, manual, or FAQ. There is also no primary academic reference to the software, but it has been used in several studies involving GIF [16–19]. From the software itself, you can write to the author's email, who declares that he is open to suggestions and comments.

When you open the program, the main screen appears with a large blank field and eight sections in the menu bar (Fig. 8.4).

The software allows you to make GIFs and histograms, spectra, spectrograms, correlations, correlograms, and other measurements of the vocal source. It can open .wav recordings from a directory, record sound, and edit it. However, it does not

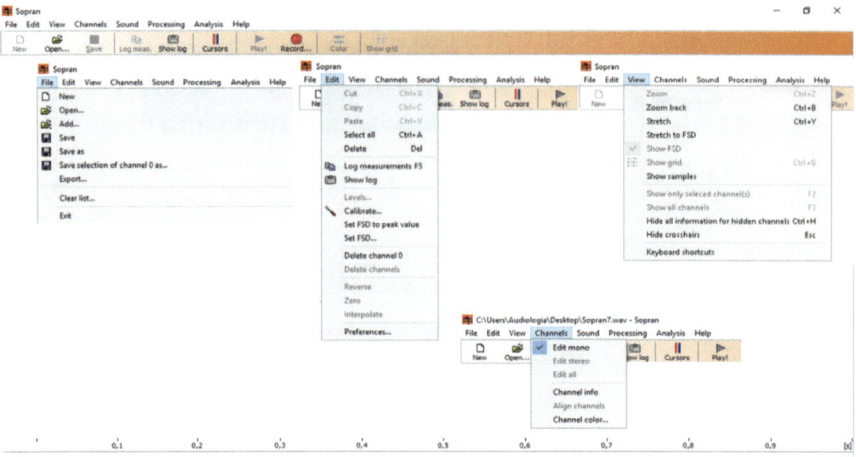

Fig. 8.4 Sopran. Sopran. The main window and the first four menus are displayed. Screenshot of Sopran, a freeware sound analysis tool developed by Tolvan Data. © Tolvan Data 2025. Used with permission

perform F0 analysis but rather a rudimentary type of zero-crossing detector. Only actions related to GIF are highlighted in this presentation.

When loading or recording audio, its waveform displays in the main window. From the *Analysis* menu, you can select the *Inverse filter* action, after which another window opens that contains the FFT of the flow, the flow derivative, and the inverses of these (Fig. 8.5), according to what is selected (as can be seen in the panel to the right of the window). In this panel, you can adjust the signal source (microphone or flow mask) in the *Home* tab and the channels in the *Make channels* tab.

If, in the Analysis menu, the action *Glottal Flow parameter measurement* is chosen instead, two panels are observed: an upper one that contains volume flow and a lower one that shows its derivative (Fig. 8.6). When you click and drag the portion of the signal you want to measure, the parameter values appear in the status bar at the bottom of the window. There, we will read the parameters' values. The log with the values can be copied and pasted using actions from the iconic menu at the top of this window. The program does not provide summary statistical measurements (mean, median, etc.) of all the signal values; only those graphically selected in the panels are used to obtain the values.

8.2.3 Online Lab Voice Clinical Systems (VCS) App

Online Lab VCS [20] is a GIF-based app for mobile devices with Android or iOS operating systems, with complementary access via the web. Its copyright belongs to *Voice Clinical Systems*, which was established in Madrid, Spain. Its principal author is Roberto Fernández-Baíllo, associate professor of engineering at the *Universidad Europea* of Madrid. It is an app that can be downloaded for free from Google Play

8 Software and Apps for Glottal Inverse Filtering   101

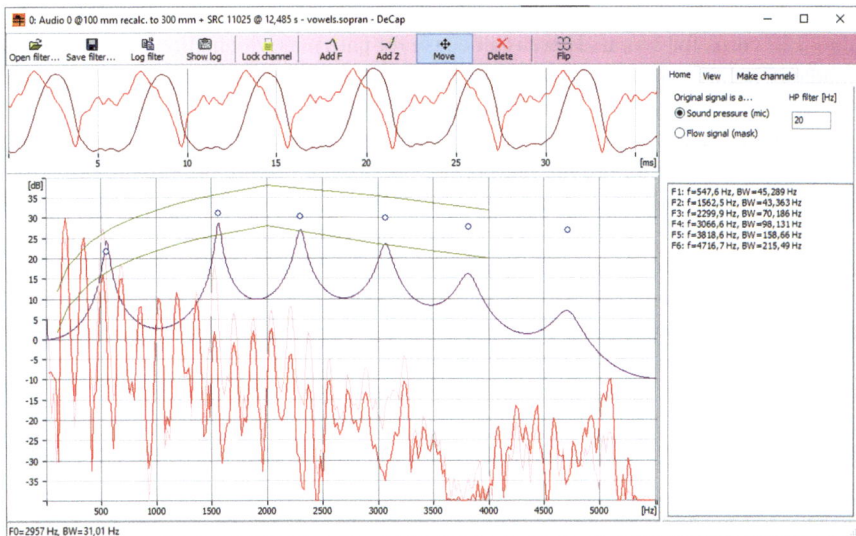

Fig. 8.5 Inverse filter. Sopran. The inverse filter window with the loaded signal is analyzed. Screenshot of Sopran, a freeware sound analysis tool developed by Tolvan Data. © Tolvan Data 2025. Used with permission

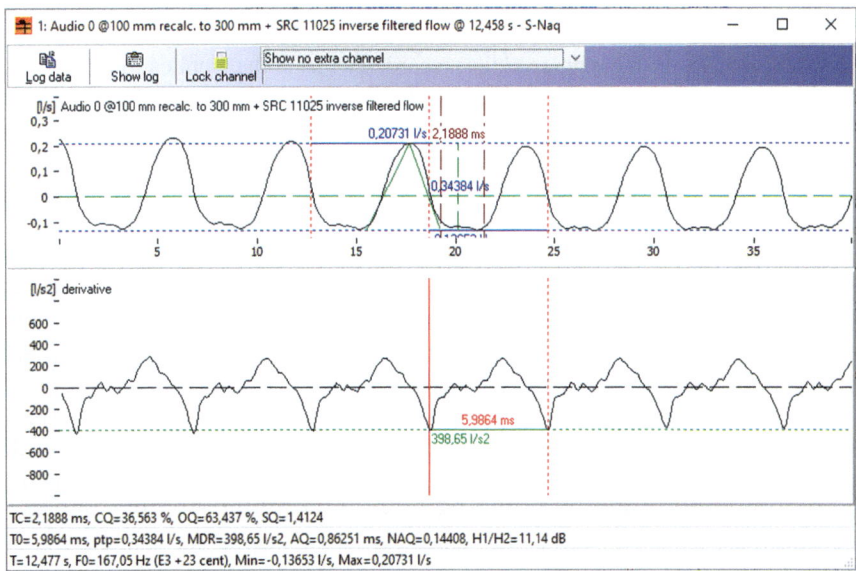

Fig. 8.6 Glottal flow parameter. Sopran. Glottal flow parameter measurement window. Screenshot of Sopran, a freeware sound analysis tool developed by Tolvan Data. © Tolvan Data 2025. Used with permission

or the App Store, but its use is available for an annual license fee for professionals—120 euros for 1 year. There is a license for patients (which allows only sending validated recordings to a registered and licensed professional of the app), and there is a license for institutions that allows up to twenty users in common with the same generated database. There is also an annual educational license that allows functions limited to screening-type reports.

The Voice Clinical Systems website is https://voiceclinicalsystems.com/, where it is possible to register and access the payment for the selected license. In addition, contact can be established with the company, and professionals can propose research projects that would receive support with a reduction in license costs and a system of discounts in the payment of the license for the presentation of research works at conferences or publications based on the use of the app.

The first version of the app, called *Online Lab*, expired at the end of 2024. The second version, which is the current one, is called *Online Lab VCS* and has several usability improvements compared to the first, although it is essentially similar. When downloading the app on a device, you must wait for the system to validate the usability of the microphone according to established standards.

For the first version, a manual was available for download from the web. In the second, the manual does not appear; instead, the website explains the details of use, the recording protocol, and a section where the biomechanical parameters are concisely explained (https://voiceclinicalsystems.com/parametros-biomecanicos/).

The interface is simple and intuitive, the functions are clearly expressed, and it is available in Spanish and English. The app captures voice recordings of one to four seconds for analysis. It cannot load files recorded with another application (Fig. 8.7).

The parameters provided by the app differ from those traditionally provided by GIF software. Although the app makes GIFs, its analyses are expressed in three different types of reports that clinically interpret the results.

The first type of report is called screening, which expresses the percentage of functional alteration and the percentage of organic alteration (injury) that is estimated to exist in the vocal cords. The second type of report is a simplified clinical test that reports estimated values for nine parameters. The third type of report is the complete clinical test that provides results for twenty-two parameters grouped into nine sets, as well as imbalance profile and dynamic profile graphs. All reports are issued in.pdf; there are no logs or exports to data sheets.

The reported categories result from the "biomechanical analysis of the vocal folds" construct, whose theoretical foundations are found in [20]. The biomechanical model integrates the theories of the mucosal wave as a traveling wave and the three-mass model of the vocal fold body-cover structure with the GIF to generate the functions and parameters. The classes and parameters are summarized in Table 8.1. Figure 8.8 shows examples of two pages of the.pdf report of an analysis carried out.

8 Software and Apps for Glottal Inverse Filtering 103

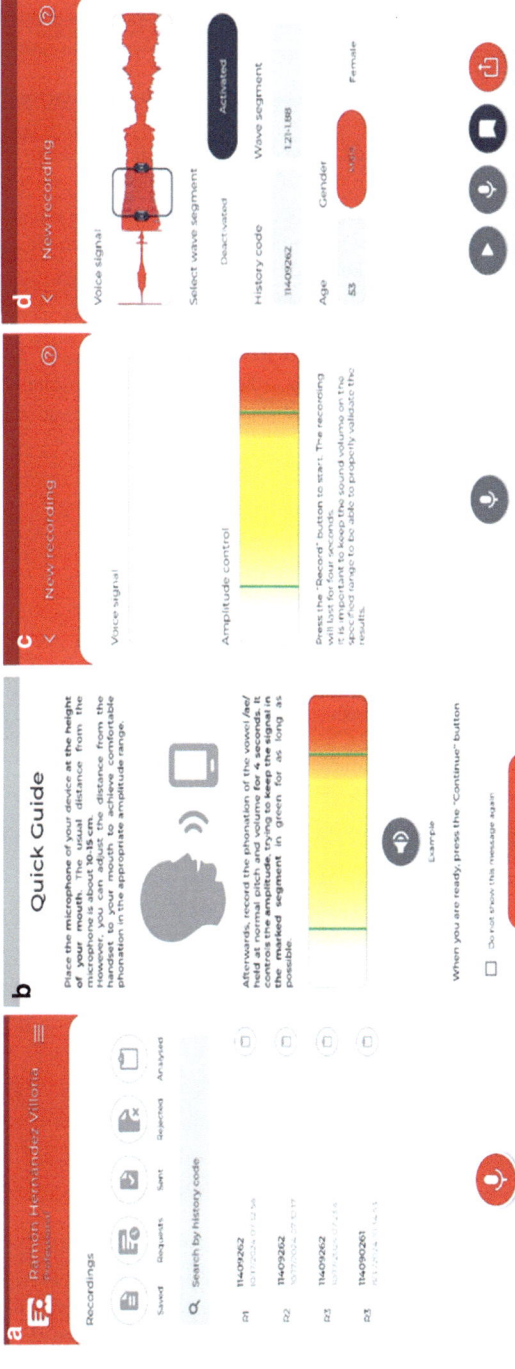

Fig. 8.7 Online Lab VCS. Capture of the four main app usage screens. (**a**). main, (**b**). quick recording guide, (**c**). recording, (**d**). capture and submit the recorded signal. Screenshot from Online Lab, © Voice Clinical Systems. Used with permission

Table 8.1 Set of parameters and parameters. Online Lab VCS. Set of parameters and parameters. r.u. = relative units

Set of parameters	Parameters
A. Fundamental frequency	F0 (Hz)
B. Vocal fold free edge harmonics movement	Ratio cycles closing (Vfa/Vfb), Asymmetry (%)
C. Phases	Closed, Open, Opening, Closing (%)
D. Muscle strength and tension	Strain Index, Closing Function Power (r.u.)
E. Sufficiency of glottal closure	Efficiency Index, Gap amplitude, Gap size (r.u.)
F. Muscle control and instability	Cycle Instability Index, Amplitude Variation Index, Vibration Blocking Index (r.u.)
G. Separation between edges (glottal amplitude)	Amplitude Index (r.u.)
H. Mucosal wave	M.W. Index closing, M.W. Index opening, Adequacy ratio M.W. closing, Adequacy ratio M.W. opening (r.u.)
I. Correlates of mass and contact alteration	Structural Imbalance Index, Mass Alteration Index (r.u.)

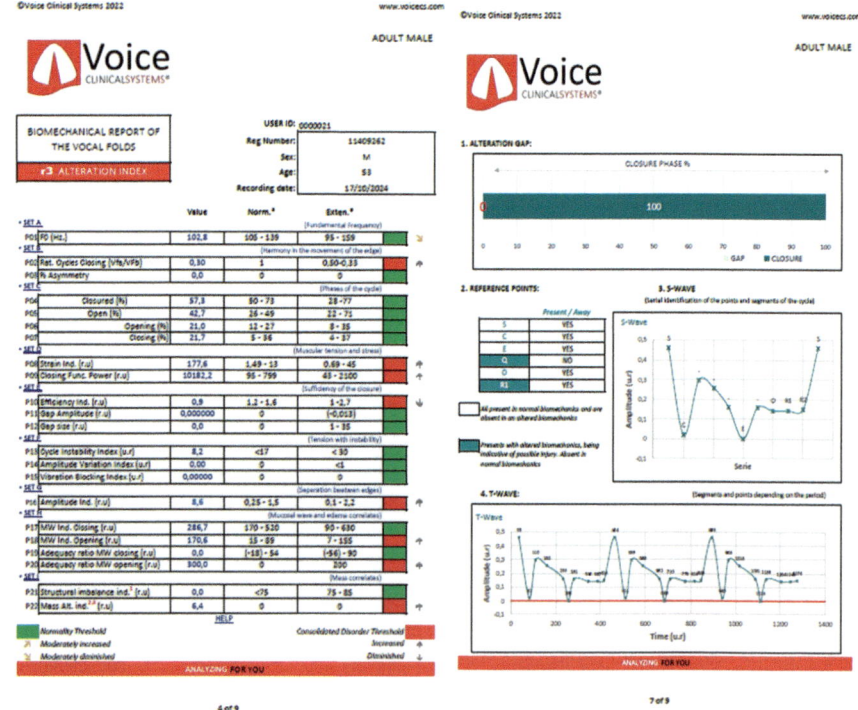

Fig. 8.8 Clinical test report for biomechanical analysis of the vocal folds. Online Lab VCS. Two-page example of a complete clinical test report for biomechanical analysis of the vocal folds. Screenshot from Online Lab, ©Voice Clinical Systems. Used with permission

8.3 Discussion

After more than five decades of development of mathematical and statistical knowledge, together with direct acoustic applications and the growing power of computational hardware, which is increasingly faster and capable of carrying out complex calculations in a few seconds, the formidable evolution of the method has been made possible. GIF and its wide range of applications in the areas of voice, both natural and artificial speech, are no exceptions. The field of interest in this volume, identifying pathologies through the approval of biomarker candidates, also has no exception.

In this chapter, two software programs and an app have been described and examined to establish their usability in the clinic. The first two, Aalto Aparat and Sopran, return parameter values. Once their meaning is understood, it is easy to know what these values indicate about the voice captured using microphones or mask flow. Although mask flow is not typical in the clinic, it is feasible in clinical research environments, and it is possible to develop more complex tools (for example, for screening) that involve using the parameters used. The two programs can also be integrated with another phoniatric clinical tool: electroglottography.

The advantages of Aalto Aparat are its user-friendliness, the robustness of algorithms, and the fact that it returns central statistical measurements over a broad signal segment. The advantages of Sopran are very similar, and another is that it allows you to record and edit the signal directly. As a common disadvantage of both programs, we can mention that they only run on Windows OS, and there are no versions for Linux OS, Chrome OS, or Mac OS. A disadvantage of Sopran is that the analysis is cycle by cycle and guided by the observer's visual judgment in deciding where the closing phase is.

Regarding Online Lab VCS, it is found that it has the virtue of taking several steps further in the evolution of specifically clinical tools for voice evaluation. This app is a solution in the mobile health field, and it is already an achievement. It runs on the two dominant mobile operating systems, iOS and Android OS, which allows for wide dissemination. On the other hand, the issue of microphone calibration and validation has been satisfactorily resolved. Another relevant aspect of this app is that it integrates the theory of the three masses in the vocal folds with the GIF method, giving practical rise to the construct of biomechanical analysis of the voice.

The expansion of the framework led to a parameterization concerned with exposing and explaining changes at the level of the vocal folds and glottis in a way that represents more concrete ideas for the clinician than the aerodynamic parameters directly offered by GIF estimation.

There are already several research references on the use of the app in areas such as vocal and laryngeal pathologies, Parkinson's Disease, Multiple Sclerosis, Amyotrophic Lateral Sclerosis (ALS), COVID-19, and in singing teaching [21–26].

The app has other advantages: although it is necessary to become familiar with its parameters, they are well represented with normal ranges. Its main disadvantage is that you must wait a few minutes for the company's server to return the result of the selected test, which is in.pdf.

8.4 Conclusions

Given their characteristics, the two PC-based software and the mobile app have great applicability in clinical and research environments in phoniatrics (intrinsic pathologies of the spoken and sung voice), laryngology, public health, and evidently as a basis for the development of voice-related biomarkers of pathologies, including neurodegenerative (Parkinson's, Alzheimer's, Huntington's, e.g.), cardiovascular, and pulmonary. They are also quite helpful in teaching singing and in the early detection of problems in at-risk educational and occupational environments.

References

1. Eysholdt U. Laryngoscopy stroboscopy, high-speed video and phonovibrogram. In: am Zehnhoff-Dinnesen A, Wiskirska-Woźnica B, Neumann K, Nawka T, editors. Phoniatrics I: fundamentals, voice disorders, disorders of language and hearing development. 1st ed. Berlin: Springer; 2020. p. 364–76. (European Manual of Medicine).
2. Herbst CT. Electroglottography – an update. J Voice. 2020 Jul;34(4):503–26. https://doi.org/10.1016/j.jvoice.2018.12.014.
3. Alku P. Glottal inverse filtering analysis of human voice production. A review of estimation and parameterization methods of the glottal excitation and their applications. Sādhanā. 2011;36(5):623–50. https://doi.org/10.1007/s12046-011-0041.
4. Alku P, Bäckström T, Vilkman E. Normalized amplitude quotient for parametrization of the glottal flow. J Acoust Soc Am. 2002 Aug;112(2):701–10. https://doi.org/10.1121/1.1490365.
5. Gobl C, Chasaide AN. Time to frequency domain mapping of the voice source: the influence of open quotient and glottal skew on the low end of the source spectrum. Interspeech. 2019;13:1961–5. https://doi.org/10.21437/interspeech.2019-2888.
6. Alku P, Strik H, Vilkman E. Parabolic spectral parameter—a new method for quantification of the glottal flow. Speech Commun. 1997;22(1):67–79. https://doi.org/10.1016/S0167-6393(97)00020-4.
7. Kreiman J, Gerratt BR, Antoñanzas-Barroso N. Measures of the glottal source spectrum. J Speech Lang Hear Res. 2007 Jun;50(3):595–610. https://doi.org/10.1044/1092-4388(2007/042).
8. Fernandes J, Teixeira F, Guedes V, Junior A, Teixeira JP. Harmonic to noise ratio measurement – Selection of window and length. Procedia Comput Sci. 2018;138:280–5. https://doi.org/10.1016/j.procs.2018.10.040.
9. Siltanen S. Glottal inverse filtering: from Stephen Hawking's voice to Siri and Alexa [Internet]. Tulane Math Colloquium; 2022 Apr 21.; Available from: https://siltanen-research.net/wp-content/uploads/talks/Tulane2022GIF_Siltanen_share.pdf. Accessed 15 Oct 2024.
10. Kafentzis G. On the (glottal) inverse filtering of speech signals [Internet]. Greece: University of Crete; 2022. Available from: https://www.csd.uoc.gr/~hy578/2022b/GIF.pdf
11. Sundberg J, Fahlstedt E, Morell A. Effects on the glottal voice source of vocal loudness variation in untrained female and male voices. J Acoust Soc Am. 2005 Feb;117(2):879–85. https://doi.org/10.1121/1.1841612.
12. Vilkman E. Occupational safety and health aspects of voice and speech professions. Folia Phoniatr Logop. 2004;56(4):220–53. https://doi.org/10.1159/000078344.
13. Pohjalainen H, Airaksinen M, Airas M, Alku P. Aalto Aparat [computer program]. Available from: http://research.spa.aalto.fi/projects/aparat/ (Retrieved and tested: 2024, October).
14. Alku P, Pohjalainen H, Airaksinen M. Aalto Aparat: a freely available tool for glottal inverse filtering and voice source parameterization. In: Proceedings of subsidia: tools and resources for speech sciences; 2017 Jun 21–23; Malaga. p. 21–23.

15. Granqvist S. Sopran [computer program]. Version 1.0.28. Tolvan Data; 2024. Available from: https://tolvan.com/index.php?page=/sopran/sopran.php (Retrieved and tested: 2024, October).
16. Kuhlmann LL, Iwarsson J. Effects of speaking rate on breathing and voice behavior. J Voice. 2024 Mar;38(2):346–56. https://doi.org/10.1016/j.jvoice.2021.09.005.
17. Lehoux S, Hampala V, Švec JG. Subglottal pressure oscillations in anechoic and resonant conditions and their influence on excised larynx phonations. Sci Rep. 2021;11(1):28. https://doi.org/10.1038/s41598-020-79265-3.
18. Strömbergsson S, Holm K, Edlund J, Lagerberg T, McAllister A. Audience response system-based evaluation of intelligibility of children's connected speech – validity, reliability and listener differences. J Commun Disord. 2020;87:106037. https://doi.org/10.1016/j.jcomdis.2020.106037.
19. Włodarczak M, Ludusan B, Sundberg J, Heldner M. Classification of voice quality using neck-surface acceleration: comparison with glottal flow and radiated sound. J Voice. 2025 Jan;39(1):10–24. https://doi.org/10.1016/j.jvoice.2022.06.034.
20. Gómez-Vilda P, Fernández-Baillo R, Nieto A, Díaz F, Fernández-Camacho FJ, Rodellar V, et al. Evaluation of voice pathology based on the estimation of vocal fold biomechanical parameters. J Voice. 2007;21(4):450–76. https://doi.org/10.1016/j.jvoice.2006.01.008.
21. Corvo-Macarro S, Solís-Rodríguez B, Fernández-Baíllo R. Estudio clínico del paciente con enfermedad de Parkinson a través del análisis biomecánico de la voz. Rev Logop Fon Audiol. 2023;43(Supl 1) 100417.2
22. Díaz Borrego P, Pérez Bonilla M, Fernández Baíllo R. Biomechanical analysis of the voice: characterization method in amyotrophic lateral sclerosis (ALS). Presented at: 51st annual symposium: care of the professional voice; 2023 May 31–June 4; Philadelphia.
23. Romero Arias T, Redondo Cortés I, Pérez Del Olmo A. Biomechanical parameters of voice in Parkinson's disease patients. Folia Phoniatr Logop. 2024;76(1):91–101. https://doi.org/10.1159/000533289.
24. Romero-Arias T, Hernández-Velasco R, Betancort M, Mena-Chamorro P, Sabater Gálvez L, Pérez Del Olmo A. Exploring biomechanical correlates in voice analysis of multiple sclerosis patients. Folia Phoniatr Logop. 2024 Jul;19:1–14. https://doi.org/10.1159/000540457.
25. Romero Arias T, Betancort MM. Voice Sequelae Following Recovery From COVID-19. J Voice. 2025 Jan;39(1):287.e19–25. https://doi.org/10.1016/j.jvoice.2022.06.033.
26. Romero-Arias T, Betancort-Montesinos M, Tari-Muntari R, Dorta-Luis J. Estudio de parámetros acústicos y biomecánicos de voz asociado a enfermedades neurodegenerativas. Rev ORL. 2018;9(7):3–6. https://doi.org/10.14201/orl.19257.

Open Access This chapter is licensed under the terms of the Creative Commons Attribution-NonCommercial-NoDerivatives 4.0 International License (http://creativecommons.org/licenses/by-nc-nd/4.0/), which permits any noncommercial use, sharing, distribution and reproduction in any medium or format, as long as you give appropriate credit to the original author(s) and the source, provide a link to the Creative Commons license and indicate if you modified the licensed material. You do not have permission under this license to share adapted material derived from this chapter or parts of it.

The images or other third party material in this chapter are included in the chapter's Creative Commons license, unless indicated otherwise in a credit line to the material. If material is not included in the chapter's Creative Commons license and your intended use is not permitted by statutory regulation or exceeds the permitted use, you will need to obtain permission directly from the copyright holder.

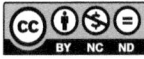

Quality Evaluation of Voice AI Software

Sneha Das

9.1 Introduction

In this chapter, we address the following question:

What constitutes sufficient evidence that a voice-AI system is clinically reliable, safe and ready for deployment?

This question extends beyond the *technical* evaluation of voice AI software, towards the discussion of the dimensions of evidence we should rely on in sensitive medical and health care applications. In other words, we address not only the performance of tools on bencmark data, but also discuss the need to consider dimensions like reliabilty of the software when interacting with patients across diverse populations, acoustic environments and recording scenarios, and mechanisms for regulatory compliance. The discussion is aimed at a) clinicians and healthcare practitioners who seek to understand what AI results imply for clinical usability, and b) developers and researchers who build voice AI software. By connecting technical evaluation to regulatory and ethical sufficiency, the chapter discusses the gap between measuring technical performance and establishing compliant clinical software, ensuring voice AI systems operate not only according to data-driven optimization, but also in accordance with values of accuracy, non-discrimination, fairness, and patient wellbeing.

The chapter is structured along three interlinked sections: Evidence from learning, ie: how data are partitioned and the learning process validated to ensure generalization beyond the training set; Evidence from performance metrics, ie: how traditional measures such as accuracy, or mean error are interpreted in clinical contexts; and Evidence from broader evaluation frameworks, ie: including regulatory oversight, clinical validation, and post-deployment monitoring that address trust, bias, and reliability over time.

S. Das (✉)
Technical University of Denmark, Kongens Lyngby, Denmark

Pioneer Centre for Artificial Intelligence, Copenhagen, Denmark
e-mail: sned@dtu.dk

9.2 Assessing the Learning Process from Data Partitioning to Reliable Generalization

The *learning process* in voice AI development can be explained as the process of determining the function that maps the input vocal biomarkers, e.g., fundamental frequency (F0), jitter, and shimmer, to the output that could be a clinical target, for instance, automatic GRBAS scoring or a Parkinson's diagnosis [1]. This mapping can be obtained through supervised learning [2], where paired examples of input and ground-truth output are used to optimize model parameters. However, the integrity of the learning process depends less on algorithmic sophistication than on how data are curated and separated for training and testing. Inadequate partitioning or unacknowledged dependencies between samples can yield deceptively high accuracy, eroding reproducibility and clinical trust. Evaluation must therefore ensure that the data organization mirrors the conditions under which the tool will ultimately be used.

9.2.1 Partitioning for Generalization

The goal of high-quality voice AI software is to perform reliably and as per expectation on the target population. The central goal of evaluation is generalization, the ability of the model to perform reliably on unseen data from the intended target population. Using an independent validation and test dataset is thus key to assessing the software for generalization and reliability, to avoid the model memorizing the training data or learning noise or undesired patterns from the data. For voice AI, this independence must be defined at multiple levels, eg: recording, speaker, session, and device. A single patient may contribute several recordings that share individual vocal idiosyncrasies; if these leak across the dataset partitions, the model may appear to detect disease while in fact recognizing the speaker. Such speaker leakage remains pervasive in published voice-health studies. When large datasets are available, they may be divided into training, validation, and test sets (Fig. 9.1). With limited data, k-fold cross-validation is commonly used, but each fold must maintain strict speaker. Beyond speaker leakage, recording channel mismatch can distort results: differences in microphones, sampling rates, or recording environments may dominate what the model learns. Similarly, task confounding, where disease and speech task covary (eg: all patients read one passage and controls another), may cause the model to learn task structure rather than pathology. Mitigating these risks requires explicit metadata tracking and, when possible, balanced experimental protocols that randomize tasks, devices, and contexts across participants. Generalization in voice AI thus depends on data independence at both the statistical and the acoustic level. Transparent reporting of how this independence is enforced should accompany any published results, as it directly determines whether performance metrics will hold when the system is deployed in real clinical environments.

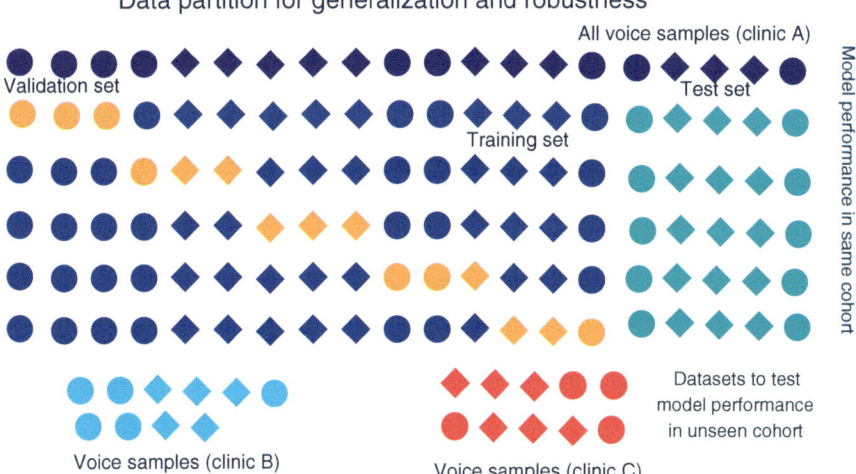

Fig. 9.1 The learning process

9.2.2 Considerations for Partitioning the Voice Samples: from Principle to Practice

The preceding discussion introduces why proper partitioning is central to assessing generalization. Yet ensuring true independence in voice AI datasets is not simply a matter of splitting data. Because the human voice encodes physiology, linguistics, and individuality simultaneously, separating 'what' from 'who' is central to the validity of voice-biomarker research. Partitioning is therefore the act by which we define what counts as generalization, and, by extension, what counts as evidence. This section translates those principles into practice, outlining the systemic considerations that govern reliable and reproducible partitioning of clinical voice data. Stratification as distributional fidelity and fairness stratification serves two purposes: preserving the distribution of diagnostic labels and ensuring equitable demographic representation. If the voice samples are divided into groups or categories, e.g., Parkinson's/no-Parkinson's, then the data partition should account for the distribution of the samples in each group, such that all the data subsets have a similar distribution of the groups. Demographic stratification ensures that performance metrics reflect genuine generalization rather than the over-representation of specific voices, languages, or recording conditions.

Cohort-based partitioning as evidence of robustness: Similar to other clinical datasets, voice datasets are often clustered around cohorts and multi-centre studies. Different cohorts (groups of patients with shared characteristics such as age, gender, region of collection or medical conditions) can display different patterns. Evaluating within and across these cohorts distinguishes models that are reproducible from those that are robust. Intra-cohort evaluation involves testing the model within a single cohort, revealing how well the software performs for that subset, for example, for female patients within a specific age group with mild Parkinson's . In contrast, inter-cohort evaluation tests whether patterns hold across contexts, eg: across clinics, languages, or time periods. This distinction parallels the difference between laboratory reproducibility and field generalization: a *voice biomarker that fails across cohorts is reliable only within its source population.*

Avoiding double dipping: Generalization requires that the test data remain completely independent from all stages of model development. In high-dimensional acoustic analysis, even subtle breaches of this independence can occur when normalization or feature selection inadvertently incorporates information from the test set. This is referred to as double-dipping or circular-analysis [3]. Such leakage transforms validation, from a test of generalization into a 'rehearsal' of the training data. Strict data isolation at every processing stage, from preprocessing to feature extraction and parameter tuning, is therefore essential (as described above and in chap. 6). Transparent documentation of partitioning boundaries and dataset provenance helps ensure that reported performance reflects genuine predictive ability.

In summary, each partitioning choice encodes an assumption about what kind of variation is meaningful and what constitutes independence, and is tied to the end goal. In this sense, the partition design is the experiment: it defines what evidence the model can legitimately provide. Without rigorous control of who speaks, when, and through what channel, even sophisticated architectures risk validating nothing more than the structure of their dataset. Few strategies for partitioning (although not exhaustive) are presented in Table 9.1.

Table 9.1 Partitioning strategies for voice AI evaluation. Each source of variability can compromise generalization if not explicitly controlled. The recommended strategies help ensure that evaluation outcomes reflect true model robustness and generalization rather than dataset artifacts

Source of variability	Risk if uncontrolled	Impact on evaluation	Recommended strategy
Speaker identity	Memorization of speaker traits	Inflated accuracy due to identity recognition	Enforce *speaker-level independence*; exclude any voice samples from the same speaker across partitions
Recording session	Leakage of temporal or contextual cues	Apparent performance gain from repeated recording conditions	Partition at the *session level* for longitudinal data; keep sessions or days strictly separate
Device or channel	Model learns recording setup instead of pathology	Poor cross-device generalization	Stratify by device type or perform *cross-device validation*; document channel conditions
Task or elicitation type	Task covaries with diagnosis (e.g., patients read different text)	Model captures task structure rather than disease signal	Balance or randomize tasks across diagnostic groups; treat task as a stratification variable
Cohort membership	Dataset-specific artifacts mistaken for generalizable features	Limited external validity; cohort bias	Conduct *intra-* and *inter-cohort* evaluations; use chronological or site-based splits to test transferability
Demographic or linguistic subgroup	Bias against underrepresented accents, genders, or age groups	Unfair or non-generalizable performance	Maintain *distributional fidelity and fairness* via stratified sampling across demographics
Temporal drift	Dataset drift across time	Model obsolescence post-deployment	Apply *chronological partitioning*; periodically re-benchmark on new data
Analytical leakage (double dipping)	Test data influence feature selection or preprocessing	Overestimated performance; circular validation	Maintain strict *data and pre-processing isolation*; document normalization and tuning procedures

9.3 Classical Evaluation Metrics

Evaluation metrics quantify how closely a model's outputs align with the intended outcomes of a given task. In voice AI systems, such metrics are indispensable for reporting performance, but their interpretation depends strongly on the type of prediction task and on the clinical context in which the system operates. Most voice AI can be categorized as performing either a classification task (eg: discrete diagnosis or screening) or a regression task (eg: continuous estimation of severity or perceptual rating). If the task is to diagnose or screen out individuals with a vocal disorder with vocal samples as input, the output would be discrete, binary, or multiclass classification, and the model will be designed as a classification task. If the task is to automatically predict the GRBAS score, a regression model would be developed, and the outcome could be continuous-valued. In this section be only briefly touch up the metrics, as there already exist exhaustive resources on this topic [2, 3].

9.3.1 Performance Metrics for Classification

Classification metrics quantify how well the software assigns instances to the correct diagnostic category (as per ground truth). In clinical voice AI applications, these metrics are used in tasks like detecting vocal biomarkers for Parkinson's disease, dysphonia and other voice pathologies. Accuracy, precision, recall, F1-score, and area under the curve (AUC) are some commonly used metrics for classification performance. Each metric captures a distinct dimension of diagnostic behavior. Accuracy reflects overall correctness but by itself can be misleading when disease prevalence is low (imbalanced datasets): if only 1% of samples represent a disorder, a model that labels every sample 'healthy' achieves 99% accuracy yet detects no true cases. In such scenarios, sensitivity, specificity, FI-score, precision provide additional insight into the diagnostic reliability of the result. The AUC summarizes the model's discrimination capacity across decision thresholds. In clinical evaluation, numerical performance must be interpreted in context. High recall with low specificity may lead to unnecessary referrals, whereas the opposite risks missed detections. Because real-world datasets often have unequal group sizes or noisy ground truth, reporting multiple complementary metrics, together with confusion matrices or receiver operating characteristic (ROC) curves, ensures transparent understanding of the trade-offs between false positives and false negatives.

9.3.2 Performance Metrics for Regression

Regression metrics assess how well a model predicts continuous outcomes, eg: perceptual ratings, measures or vocal impairment and disease progression. Common metrics are mean absolute error (MAE) and mean squared error (MSE), which measure the average magnitude or squared difference between the software output and the ground truth value. R^2, which is the coefficient of determination, measures the proportion of variance explained by the model relative to the variance explained by the mean. Values close to 1.0 indicate better model fit. Many clinical scales are ordinal or quasi-continuous rather than strictly interval-scaled, ie: their numeric steps are ordered but not guaranteed to represent equal perceptual differences. Inter-rater variability can aid set an upper bound on achievable R^2. Consequently, reporting inter-rater reliability (or variability) alongside model performance provides critical context for what constitutes a 'good' prediction. Additionally, error-based metrics should be interpreted relative to clinically meaningful thresholds, for instance, whether MAE < 0.5 corresponds to a distinguishable difference on the GRBAS scale, to help convey the practical implications of model performance.

Note: Classical evaluation metrics offer valuable performance insights, but their clinical relevance depends on careful interpretation. For voice AI systems, the optimal evaluation approach often involves combining multiple metrics, conducting an error analysis, and aligning performance thresholds with clinical priorities. By integrating these metrics with real-world validation strategies, researchers can build voice AI tools that not only perform well technically but also deliver meaningful clinical impact.

9.4 From Performance Sufficiency to Trustworthy Evidence

The previous chapters demonstrated how voice biomarkers and AI software hold significant potential in healthcare for scalable voice disorder monitoring and management, and the previous sections in this chapter discussed the technical assessment of models. However, the clinical readiness of AI relies not only on technical performance metrics but also on regulatory frameworks and operational standards. In the following section, we briefly discuss these additional factors on regulatory oversight and clinical trials toward ensuring the safety, reliability, and efficacy of voice-AI tools.

9.4.1 Regulation as a Foundation for Trust in Healthcare

Regulatory frameworks provide the governance scaffolding necessary to ensure voice AI tools meet the safety, efficacy, and ethical requirements of the tools deployed in healthcare and other high-stakes applications. The EU Artificial Intelligence Act (2024) [4] classifies medical AI as high risk, mandating human oversight, transparency of model behavior, and post-market surveillance. Further, the International Medical Device Regulators Forum's (IMDRF) *Good Machine Learning Practice principles* [5] and the WHO *Ethics and Governance of Artificial Intelligence for Health report* [6] emphasize accountability, traceability, and equity as cornerstones of trustworthy AI. Regulatory adherence enables researchers to think beyond quantitative performance, in terms of accuracy, and to incorporate broader assessment metrics like clinical interpretability, bias, and reliability audits over time. Across these frameworks, evaluation is increasingly viewed as an evidence collection across AI-lifecycle comprising three complementary stages [7, 8]: a) Preclinical (technical) validation, using technical metrics discussed above, demonstrates the software's accuracy and robustness on retrospective datasets. b) Clinical validation would reflect clinical utility through prospective studies, and

c) post-deployment monitoring of deployed systems will aid in real-world performance degradation or unforeseen adverse events. However, within the sphere of voice software employing AI technology for use in medical and clinical settings, the exact roadmap from preclinical development to post-deployment validation is an open (research) question yet to be operationalized. Current frameworks that claim to operationalize regulatory compliance are largely modality-agnostic and provide no explicit criteria for evaluating acoustic robustness, accent or language fairness, or resilience to safety and security threats to the AI software, like voice spoofing and re-identification. While these frameworks are great starting points, they may not translate directly to voice, whose biometric nature and dependence on uncontrolled acoustic conditions, speaking behavior, and linguistic diversity introduce privacy, security, and fairness challenges not encountered in standardized imaging or laboratory data. Defining how these general regulatory principles translate into domain-specific evaluation procedures is therefore essential for operational trust in voice AI.

9.4.2 RCTs and Beyond for Voice AI

Randomized controlled trials (RCTs) remain the gold standard for establishing causal relationships between interventions and outcomes. In principle, voice AI tools could be evaluated through RCTs that randomize participants to receive standard care versus AI-augmented care, such as AI-assisted Parkinson's screening, or through cross-over and cluster designs comparing AI-supported and conventional workflows at the patient or clinic level [9, 10]. Despite their conceptual appeal, RCTs evaluating AI interventions remain uncommon. Recent reviews identified only a few dozen such studies among thousands screened, with most limited to small, single-center evaluations and narrow clinical endpoints [10]. The trials that do exist also show recurrent methodological weaknesses. Systematic assessments have reported incomplete descriptions of how the AI system was trained, updated, or integrated into clinical workflow, as well as limited transparency around data handling and human oversight [11]. There are also feasibility challenges: AI systems, including voice-based systems, are adaptive. They may change as new data are encountered, they can depend on recording context (microphone type, noise environment, speaking style), and they can actively shape clinician decision-making. These properties strain traditional RCT assumptions about having a fixed, stable 'intervention' blinding, and reproducibility across sites [12]. In traditional systems these factors mainly introduce measurement noise that can be statistically controlled or averaged out. In AI-driven systems, by contrast, variability actively shapes model behavior, the system learns from and adapts to the very conditions that cause it. This coupling between data source and model makes reproducibility and control more difficult to achieve within conventional trial frameworks.

Formal reporting frameworks have begun to emerge. The CONSORT-AI and SPIRIT-AI extensions provide structured guidance for how to design and report clinical trials that evaluate AI interventions, including requirements to describe the AI system, how input data are acquired, how the model interacts with clinicians, and how its outputs influence care pathways [13]. For earlier-stage, live clinical testing of AI decision-support systems, the DECIDE-AI guideline proposes a checklist of items that should be reported when introducing an AI tool into real clinical workflows for the first time [14]. These efforts make evaluation more transparent and comparable across studies. However, adherence to these frameworks is still inconsistent [11], and they were not developed with voice as a primary input modality. As mentioned earlier, voice AI introduces sources of variability, that are rarely controlled in trials, but that directly affect model outputs. This means that we will have to develop methods and frameworks to account for the the uncontrolled acoustic scenarios of remote monitoring, telehealth, or home use.

9.4.3 Towards a Standard of Necessary and Sufficient Evidence for Voice AI

Defining sufficient evidence for the safety and clinical validity of voice AI remains an open challenge. Conventional evaluation and metrics discussed in chapter 6 and in the above sections, quantify algorithmic performance. Additional assessment dimensions and frameworks are necessary to establish the safety and reliability of the system in practice. For medical AI, sufficiency must integrate quantitative performance with demonstrable clinical benefit, interpretability, and sustained reliability across populations and contexts [6, 13, 14]. A dedicated evaluation guideline for voice AI, comparable to those for imaging [3] or genomic AI is yet to be developed. Developing such standards will require coordinated input from cross-disciplinary experts, like clinicians, signal-processing and ML experts, and regulators to translate existing general frameworks into voice-specific requirements. Building on emerging trustworthy-AI frameworks, evidence for voice AI can be understood through three interdependent dimensions [4, 6, 13, 14]: a) technical robustness b) clinical utility c) ethical and social alignment. To operationalize the voice AI framework, we can begin with the following infrastructural and research development 1) Benchmarking: develop shared audio and voice datasets which are annotated and reflect device, language and demographic diversity. Similar to the role of ImageNet in vision research, a 'VoiceNet-Health' repository could serve as a reproducibility anchor. 2) Data- and model-sheets: Adopt structured reporting templates, building on MINIMAR [7] and CONSORT-AI [13], to record model lineage, data provenance, and update policies. Such documentation should accompany regulatory submissions under the EU AI Act [4]. 3) Post-deployment monitoring: develop continuous surveillance of model drift and fairness, using automatically logged acoustic statistics and demographic performance audits. Thresholds for retraining or rollback should be pre-specified (or pre-registered) and auditable by non-conflicted third-parties.

Voice AI thus calls for going beyond one-off validation, *towards a continuous and adaptable evidence-generating ecosystem*. Operational sufficiency is a step closer to feasibility when technical benchmarking, clinical testing, and ethical auditing are institutionalized as routine components of development and regulation.

9.5 Summary

Evaluating voice AI software requires moving from accuracy-centered validation toward sufficiency of evidence across technical, clinical, and ethical dimensions. Reliable learning, robust performance, and alignment with regulatory and human values together determine whether a system is ready for clinical integration. Voice-related biomarkers, being inherently sensitive and variable, demand transparency in data handling and continuous post-deployment evaluation. Future efforts should establish standardized voice-specific evaluation protocols, ensuring that these technologies remain not only effective but also safe, fair, and trustworthy.

References

1. Hidaka S, Lee Y, Nakanishi M, Wakamiya K, Nakagawa T, Kaburagi T. Automatic GRBAS scoring of pathological voices using deep learning and a small set of labelled voice data. J Voice. 2022;S0892-1997(22):00347-2. https://doi.org/10.1016/j.jvoice.2022.10.020.
2. Hardt M, Recht B. Patterns, predictions, and actions: a story about machine learning. arXiv preprint arXiv:2102.05242. 2021. https://fairmlbook.org/pdf/patterns.pdf, https://mlstory.org/.
3. Olivier C. Machine learning for brain disorders. New York: Springer US; 2023. https://library.oapen.org/handle/20.500.12657/75361.
4. Veale M, Zuiderveen BF. Demystifying the draft EU artificial intelligence act—Analysing the good, the bad, and the unclear elements of the proposed approach. Comput Law Rev Int. 2021;22(4):97–112.
5. US Food and Drug Administration. Good machine learning practice for medical device development. US Food and Drug Administration [Internet]; 2021. https://www.fda.gov/medical-devices/software-medical-device-samd/good-machine-learning-practice-medical-device-development-guiding-principles.
6. World Health Organization. Ethics and governance of artificial intelligence for health: large multi-modal models. WHO guidance. World Health Organization; 2024. https://www.who.int/publications/i/item/9789240084759.
7. Hernandez-Boussard T, Bozkurt S, Ioannidis JPA, Shah NH. MINIMAR (MINimum Information for Medical AI Reporting): Developing reporting standards for artificial intelligence in health care. J Am Med Inform Assoc. 2020;27(12):2011-5. https://doi.org/10.1093/jamia/ocaa088.
8. Morley J, Machado CCV, Burr C, Cowls J, Joshi I, Taddeo M, et al. The ethics of AI in health care: A mapping review. Soc Sci Med. 2020;260:113172. https://doi.org/10.1016/j.socscimed.2020.113172.
9. Han R, Acosta JN, Shakeri Z, Ioannidis JPA, Topol EJ, Rajpurkar P. Randomised controlled trials evaluating artificial intelligence in clinical practice: a scoping review. Lancet Digit Health. 2024 May;6(5):e367–73. https://doi.org/10.1016/S2589-7500(24)00047-5.
10. Thomas Y T, Lam Max F K, Cheung Yasmin L, Munro Kong Meng, Lim Dennis, Shung Joseph J Y, Sung (2022) Randomized Controlled Trials of Artificial Intelligence in Clinical Practice: Systematic Review Journal of Medical Internet Research 24(8) e37188-10.2196/37188
11. Shahzad R, Ayub B, Siddiqui MAR. Quality of reporting of randomised controlled trials of artificial intelligence in healthcare: a systematic review. BMJ Open. 2022;12(9) e061519. 10.1136/bmjopen-2022-061519.

12. DavidChen D, Cao C, Kloosterman R, Parsa R, Raman S. Trial factors associated with zompletion of clinical trials evaluating AI: retrospective case-control study. J Med Internet Res. 2024;26e58578. 10.2196/58578.
13. Liu X, Cruz Rivera S, Moher D, Calvert MJ, Denniston AK, Andrew HA, et al. Reporting guidelines for clinical trial reports for interventions involving artificial intelligence: the CONSORT-AI extension. Lancet Digit Health. 2020;2(10):e537-e548. https://doi.org/10.1016/S2589-7500(20)30218-1.
14. Baptiste, Vasey Myura, Nagendran Bruce, Campbell David A, Clifton Gary S, Collins Spiros, Denaxas Alastair K, Denniston Livia, Faes Bart, Geerts Mudathir, Ibrahim Xiaoxuan, Liu Bilal A, Mateen Piyush, Mathur Melissa D, McCradden Lauren, Morgan Johan, Ordish Campbell, Rogers Suchi, Saria Daniel S W, Ting Peter, Watkinson Wim, Weber Peter, Wheatstone Peter, McCulloch Reporting guideline for the early stage clinical evaluation of decision support systems driven by artificial intelligence: DECIDE-AI BMJ e070904-10.1136/bmj-2022-070904.

Open Access This chapter is licensed under the terms of the Creative Commons Attribution-NonCommercial-NoDerivatives 4.0 International License (http://creativecommons.org/licenses/by-nc-nd/4.0/), which permits any noncommercial use, sharing, distribution and reproduction in any medium or format, as long as you give appropriate credit to the original author(s) and the source, provide a link to the Creative Commons license and indicate if you modified the licensed material. You do not have permission under this license to share adapted material derived from this chapter or parts of it.

The images or other third party material in this chapter are included in the chapter's Creative Commons license, unless indicated otherwise in a credit line to the material. If material is not included in the chapter's Creative Commons license and your intended use is not permitted by statutory regulation or exceeds the permitted use, you will need to obtain permission directly from the copyright holder.

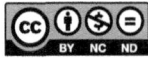

Part II

Clinical Applications

Pathology of Voice-Related Biomarkers in Laryngology

10

Neveen Hassan Nashaat

10.1 Introduction

Voice-related biomarkers are features related to voice that have been identified as associated with clinical outcomes. They can be used to diagnose a condition, grade the severity, and identify the stages of a voice disorder, or they can be used for management and follow-up. Biomarkers could be diagnostic, monitoring, response, predictive, prognostic, susceptibility, or complex biomarkers [1]. For example, the auditory perceptual assessment of dysphonia and the glottic closure pattern were reported to be predictors of the voice therapy sessions number. Moreover, the hourglass pattern of glottic closure predicted a longer duration of intervention in laryngeal edema or benign vocal fold lesions [2]. The voice quality is influenced by a variety of laryngeal disorders, including organic and non-organic disorders, in addition to minimal associated pathological lesions (MAPLs) [e.g., nodules, polyps, and Reinke's edema]. Disorders affecting only the voice box or other body systems, including the larynx, lead to pathological changes in voice-related biomarkers.

The European Laryngological Society and the Union of European Phoniatricians have suggested statements or guidelines for baseline evaluations and pre- and post-treatment assessments of voice quality, which could be used as biomarkers. They included clinical measures, clinical diagnostic aids, and additional instrumental measures [3, 4]. Other measures have also been reported in the literature to compensate for certain requirements in commonly used instruments, including cepstral analysis of voice, some measures of electroglottography, maximum flow declination rate, and inverse filtering [5, 6]. The contribution of the different disorders in the change of voice (dysphonia) and how they influence voice quality and laryngeal functions differs. The pathology of voice-related biomarkers is discussed in this chapter for some laryngological disorders other than neurogenic ones.

N. H. Nashaat (✉)
Research on Children with Special Needs Department, Medical Research and Clinical Studies Institute, National Research Centre, Cairo, Egypt

© The Author(s) 2026
M. Pedersen et al. (eds.), *Voice-related Biomarkers*,
https://doi.org/10.1007/978-3-032-03134-1_10

10.2 Perspectives Regarding Voice-Related Biomarkers

10.2.1 Auditory Perceptual Assessment

It is used to comment on the voice quality using scales that were developed by voice experts for the diagnosis and follow-up of pathological voices, such as the GRBAS scale concerning the grading of *severity, roughness, and breathiness, in addition to asthenia and strain*, or the modified GRBAS scale developed by Kotby [4], including the grade, character, pitch, *register*, loudness, glottal attack, and comments on associated laryngeal functions (e.g., cough). *The grades given* in *these systems are mild (1), moderate (2), and severe (3). Grade 0 is given for a normal or nondysphonic voice.* The Consensus Auditory Perceptual Evaluation of Voice (CAPE-V) scale uses a 100-point grading of strain, roughness, and breathiness. It includes pitch and loudness, together with comments on resonance and features of voice (e.g., tremors, gurgling). A correlation was found between this scale and the modified GRBAS [7].

As reported by Kotby [4], *the character of the voice* could be strained, leaky, breathy, or irregular. In hyperfunctional voice disorders, where muscular tension is high, a strained, leaky character is usually heard. A strained voice is usually characterized by a stronger second harmonic than the first one, with a long period of glottal closure during vibration [8]. A breathy voice is commonly noticed in unilateral vocal fold (VF) immobility or scarring where the size of the gap is large. Air escape could be associated with high subglottic pressure to increase the loudness. Irregular characteristics could be noticed in MAPLs or functional and organic voice disorders, such as laryngeal changes in endocrine disorders (e.g., hypothyroidism). It could be heard as a result of VF asymmetry in mass or tension. Irregularity could be perceived when the stiffness of the cover layer is significantly reduced while maintaining the same level of subglottic pressure. Furthermore, a glottal gap could lead to an irregular voice character [9].

Changes in the pitch could be detected in a variety of laryngeal pathologies. It could be reduced in MAPLs or diplophonic in mutational voice disorders. The pitch range is commonly reduced in thyroid gland dysfunction [10]. The voice pitch is modulated primarily by the fine changes in the VF tension. The greater stiffness or tension in the VFs makes them vibrate at a high frequency during phonation. Stiffness is a property of the VF representing the force of elastic restoration in response to deformation. The VF stress or tension describes its mechanical state [12]. Furthermore, a reduction in the VF length leads to a change in pitch [13]. Commenting on the register includes falsetto, head, chest, or modal, along with the presence of register breaks. Falsetto register could be observed in some cases with unilateral VF immobility [11]. When someone attempts to increase the fundamental frequency (F0) by increasing the cricothyroid activation alone, the VFs, with a small thickness of the medial surface, reduced maximum flow declination rate, and a brief duration of glottal closure, are prepared to produce a falsetto voice (Fig. 10.1). The falsetto voice occurs with nearly sinusoidal flow waveforms, incomplete glottic closure, and a limited number of harmonics [12]. A falsetto register occurs when the

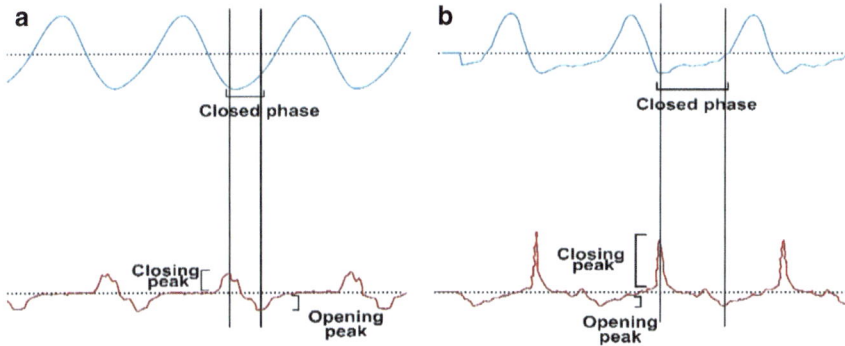

Fig. 10.1 Graphical changes of registers. Change in CT activation leading to a shorter closed phase to produce (**a**) falsetto register; the closed phase and closing peak are shorter compared to (**b**) the modal register; there is no change in the opening peak

voice is at the higher end of the pitch range. In conversational speech, the modal voice is produced with an intermediate thickness of the VF at the intermediate range of pitch. Vocal fry is produced with increased vertical thickness and a long duration of glottic closure. It occurs at the lower end of the pitch range [14].

Reduced or fluctuating loudness is usually seen in laryngeal pathologies, e.g., hyperthyroidism, hypofunctional dysphonia, sulcus vocalis, and VF immobility. Attempting to increase the voice intensity is associated with high subglottic pressure, together with the high duration of the closed phase of the VF vibration cycle [15].

The presence of a hard glottal attack, which is the vocal behavior of hard voice onset, can be observed with hyperfunctional dysphonia and MAPLs [16]. It results from tight glottic closure, more adduction strength of the VF, and compression of supraglottic structures. It is associated with greater voice onset time, phonation threshold pressure, and shimmer values when compared with the voice parameters of those who do not have a hard glottal attack [17].

Assessment of associated laryngeal functions, such as cough, whispers, and laughter, is essential, considering they are influenced by some laryngeal lesions, including disorders causing VF immobility; on the other hand, chronic cough could lead to dysphonia [18].

10.2.2 Videolaryngostroboscopy and/or High-Speed Films

The visualization of the larynx using videolaryngostroboscopy helps clinicians to judge mucosal wave symmetry, amplitude, morphology, and movements.

Mucosal wave symmetry

Asymmetry of the mucosal wave occurs in unilateral VF lesions, including MAPLs, or in bilateral asymmetric lesions, such as leukoplakia or Reinke's edema.

Amplitude of the mucosal wave

It could be normal, mild, moderate, or severely decreased. The amplitude is decreased when the medial margins of the VFs mucosa move laterally less than one-third of the width of the VFs. Reduced mucosal wave vibrations have been reported in MAPLs, non-organic dysphonia (e.g., hyperfunctional dysphonia), VF dehydration, VF scars, and sulcus vocalis [19].

Morphology

Comments on the morphology of the whole larynx area during breathing and phonation, along with the lesion and laryngeal disorder when present, are essential. In Leukoplakia, non-homogenous color, irregular texture, prominent thickness, vascularization perpendicular to the lesion, and vessel loops predicted malignancy [19]. Adduction of the supraglottal structures, which is often observed in muscle tension dysphonia, may lead to mediolateral or anteroposterior constriction of the airway, which is immediately above the VFs [20]. Masses of the VF should be described regarding the site, size, shape, surface, and mucosal wave over the mass. Figure 10.2 shows different shapes of VF masses (mostly laryngeal tumors), whereas Fig. 10.3 shows the forms of VF webs.

Movements

VF movement, ventricular fold contribution, and glottal closure patterns (complete, incomplete, anterior gap, posterior gap, irregular, or hourglass) should be observed [21]. The contribution of the ventricular fold to phonation results from the underlying VF pathology. The glottic gap (phonatory gap or phonatory waste) could result from changes in VF mass, VF tension, or the presence of lesions [9]. Figure 10.4 shows anterior and posterior glottal gaps and incomplete glottic closure. Figure 10.5 shows an hourglass glottal gap. Figure 10.6 shows the fusiform gap of the VF. Figure 10.7 shows an irregular glottal gap attributed to different pathologies.

10.2.3 Patient-Reported Voice Quality Assessment

There are scales that are used for voice-related quality of life. The 30- or 10-version of the Voice Handicap Index (VHI) are validated scales in many languages and different populations (Table 10.1) [22]. The scores of these scales are high in laryngeal pathology. The VHI was reported to improve after voice therapy measures. The functional subscale of the VHI was reported to be correlated with the NHR in MAPLs [23].

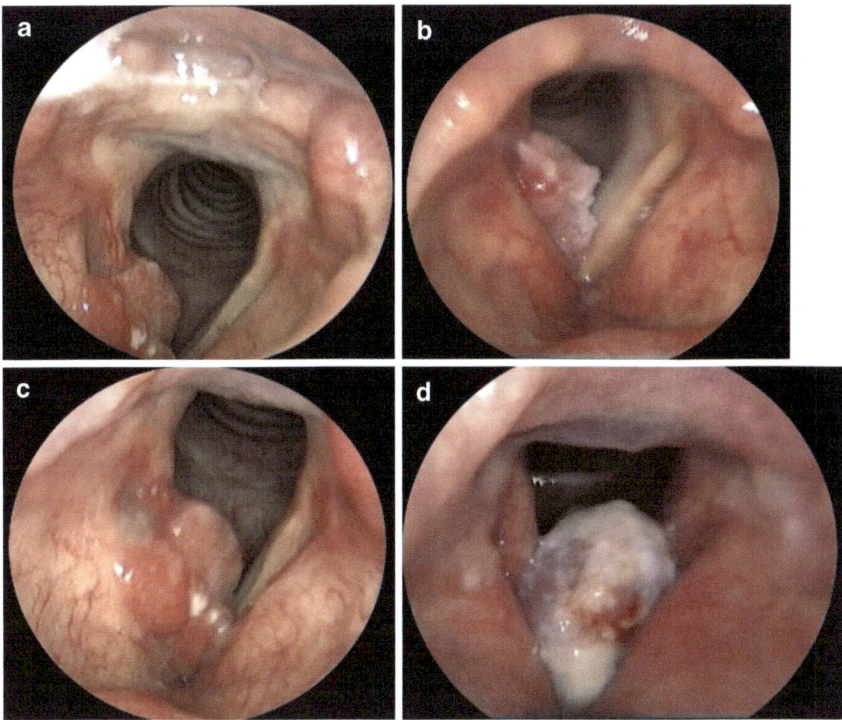

Fig. 10.2 Different shapes of VF mass. Different shapes of VF mass: (**a**) Irregular mass of the anterior half of the right VF; (**b**) Irregular mass of the right VF; (**c**) Irregular mass of the right VF; (**d**) Irregular mass of the left VF

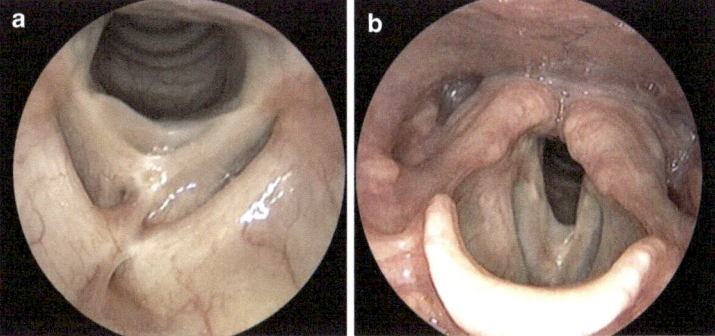

Fig. 10.3 Different shapes of acquired VF web. Different shapes of acquired VF web: (**a**) involving the VF length; (**b**) involving the majority of the VF length

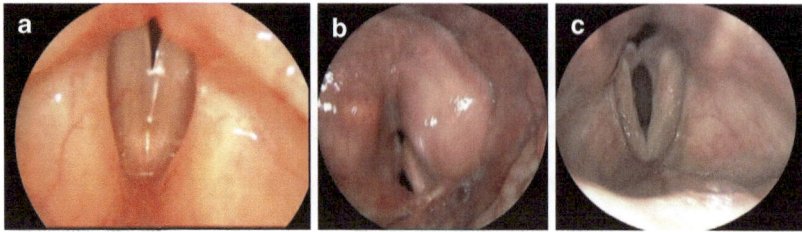

Fig. 10.4 Examples of phonatory gap patterns during phonation. Phonatory gap patterns during phonation: (**a**) posterior glottal gap; (**b**) anterior glottal gap attributed to right VF scar; (**c**) incomplete glottic closure leading to double gap

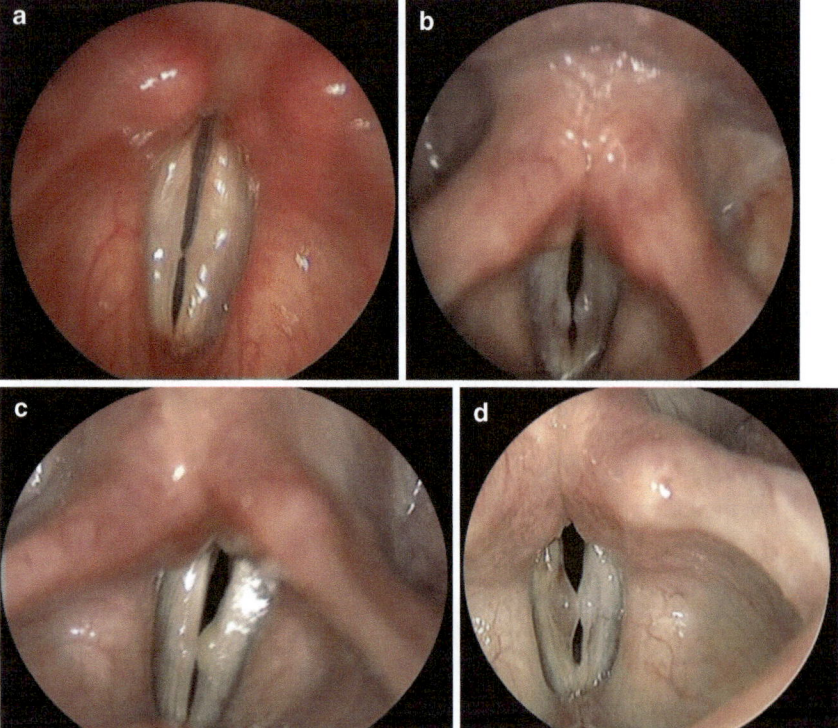

Fig. 10.5 The hourglass glottal gap during phonation, The hourglass glottal gap during phonation: (**a**) Early bilateral VF nodules; (**b**) Bilateral VF nodules; (**c**) Left VF cyst; (**d**) Right VF cyst with left VF reaction

10 Pathology of Voice-Related Biomarkers in Laryngology

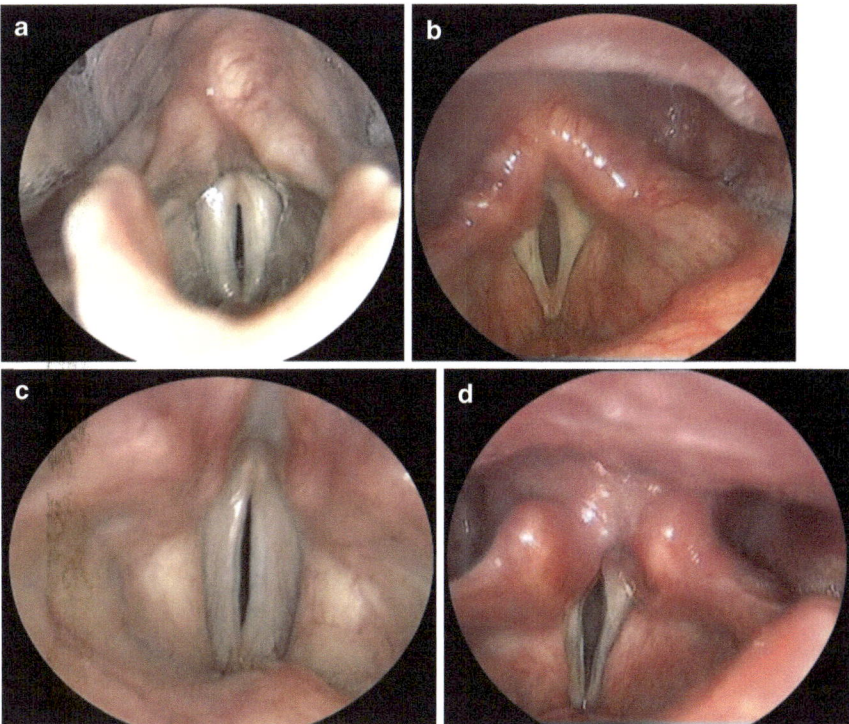

Fig. 10.6 Fusiform glottal gap during phonation. Fusiform glottal gap during phonation with different types of laryngeal pathology: (**a**) Fusiform phonatory gap in a case with early Parkinson's disease; (**b**) Fusiform phonatory gap in a case with advanced Parkinson's disease; (**c**) Fusiform phonatory gap with right VF sulcus vocalis; (**d**) Fusiform phonatory gap with bilateral sulcus vocalis

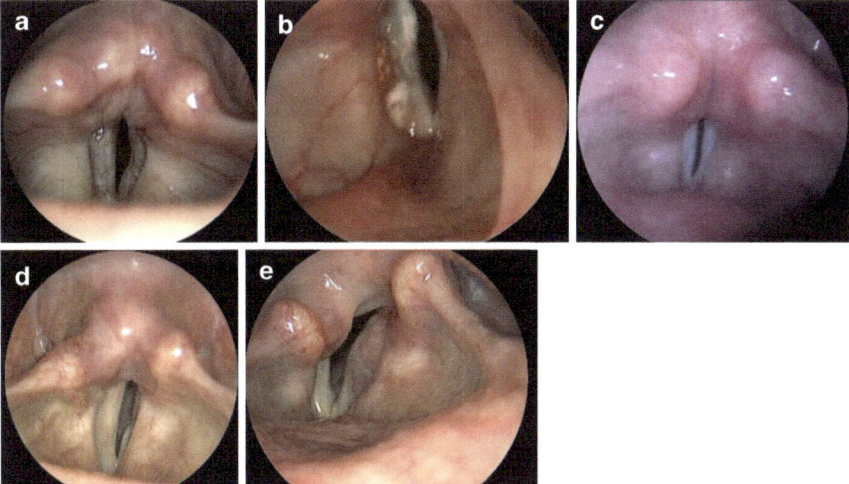

Fig. 10.7 Irregular glottal gap during phonation. Irregular glottal gap during phonation attributed to different laryngeal pathologies: (**a**) Left VF scar; (**b**) Right VF scar; (**c**) Left VF scar; (**d**) Left VF posterior cordectomy; (**e**) Irregular phonatory gap attributed to multiple laryngeal pathologies

Table 10.1 Voice Handicap Index—10 questions. Shows the Voice Handicap Index test of subjective complaints with 10 questions

Voice Handicap Index (VHI-10)	
How to complete this questionnaire:	
These are statements many people have used to describe their voices and the effects of their voices on their lives.	
Please circle the response that indicates how frequently you have the same experience.	
0–4 rating scale	
0 = never	
1 = almost never	
2 = sometimes	
3 = almost always	
4 = always	
Situation	*Frequency of problem*
My voice makes it difficult for people to hear me	0 1 2 3 4
People have difficulty understanding me in a noisy room	0 1 2 3 4
My voice difficulties restrict my personal and social life	0 1 2 3 4
I feel left out of the conversations because of my voice.	0 1 2 3 4
My voice problem causes me to lose income.	0 1 2 3 4
I feel as though I have to strain to produce my voice	0 1 2 3 4
The clarity of my voice is unpredictable.	0 1 2 3 4
My voice problem upsets me	0 1 2 3 4
My voice makes me feel handicapped	0 1 2 3 4
People ask, "what's wrong with your voice?"	0 1 2 3 4
TOTAL	

10.2.4 Acoustic Analysis

Acoustic analysis is mostly performed using a computer program, which quantitatively elucidates several measurable aspects of the captured voice signals, such as the mean fundamental frequency (F0), shimmer, jitter, and noise-to-harmonics ratio (NHR), which are widely used measures (Fig. 10.8). The intensity of the sounds could influence the results of the acoustic analysis. Therefore, patients could be under their own control. It can be possibly performed at different levels of 60, 70, and 80 dB. It is advised to be performed on pronouncing the sustained vowel /a/. The 3 middle seconds on the same decibel level should be considered with the microphone placed 4 cm from the mouth. Additional acoustic measurements should be included in the assessment of voice quality for voice professionals: standard deviation of F0, minimal intensity (dB), maximal intensity (dB), and range of intensity (dB) [3]. It could be performed by Praat software and VOX plot, which are freely available, or the multidimensional voice program [24, 25]. Jitter and shimmer were reported to be influenced by the selected vowel for analysis and the phonation frequency. Furthermore, these measures cannot be obtained in cases of severe dysphonia with high aperiodicity. Cepstral analysis was reported to be used to overcome the limitations of these time-based measures [26].

Fundamental Frequency (F0)

F0 is the first harmonic, representing the number of glottic cycles that the VFs perform in one second. It is measured in hertz (Hz). It depends on the length, depth, thickness, stress, and stiffness conditions of the VFs. It could be reduced in many organic, MAPLs, and non-organic voice disorders or raised in other disorders (mutational). F0 increases with low length and higher stiffness and stress. Moreover, F0 rises by increasing the contact time of VF and higher subglottic pressure [12].

Jitter

Jitter is the periodic (duration) variation from cycle to cycle. The voices of individuals with laryngeal pathologies usually have a higher percentage of jitter. This is related to the lack of VF vibration control. Furthermore, it was reported to be correlated with the size of a VF polyp [24].

Shimmer

This represents the amplitude variation of the waves in the voice. In voice disorders, the percentage of shimmer increases. The shimmer changes with the reduction of glottic resistance and the presence of mass lesions on the VFs, and it has a relation with the presence of breathiness.

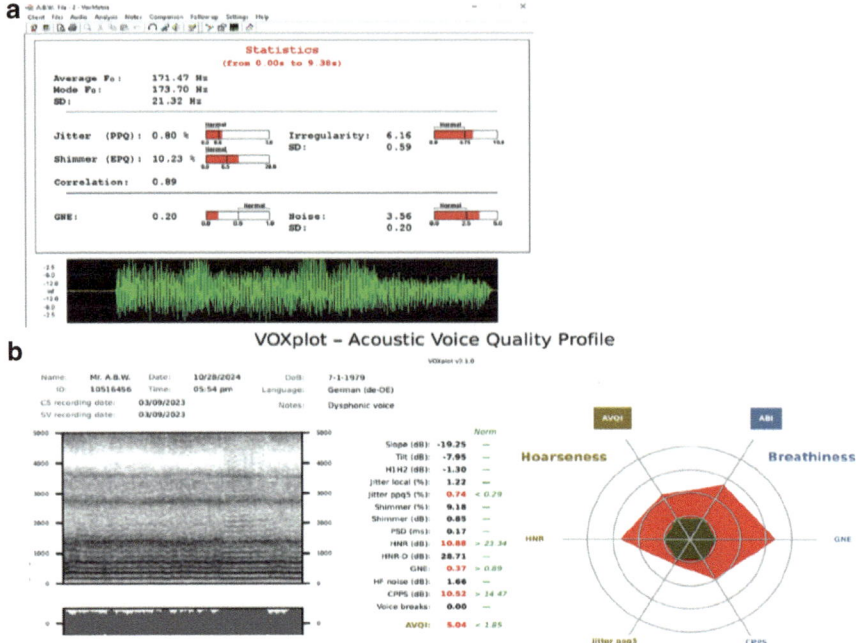

Fig. 10.8 VOXplot acoustic analysis of voice samples for patients with dysphonia. Different outcomes of acoustic analysis of voice samples from patients with dysphonia: (**a**) sF0, jitter, and shimmer; (**b**) more parameters with a graphical representation of voice. Screenshot of VOXplot licensed under the GNU General Public License v3 (GPLv3). © lingphon/Jörg Mayer. The GNU General Public License v3 can be found at https://www.gnu.org/licenses/gpl-3.0.html

Noise to Harmonics Ratio (NHR)

NHR is the ratio between the non-periodic and periodic components of the voice. It is measured in decibels (dB). It was reported to increase in many voice disorders. Breathiness and roughness of voice were correlated with the NHR [27]. It was found to be a more sensitive indicator of vocal function than jitter for assessment of the aging voice [28].

Cepstrum

The cepstrum is a Fourier transform representation of the logarithmic magnitude of the spectrum. Cepstral analysis is an acoustic analysis measure used to quantify F0 and harmonic organization in the voice. Cepstral Peak Prominence (CPP) estimates additive noise or aperiodicity without identification of cycle boundaries. Therefore, it can be identified in connected speech, as well as in sustained vowel productions [5]. The periodic voice signal will have a high amplitude of CPP (dB). A low-amplitude CPP represents a weakly periodic or aperiodic voice signals [29]. The objective comparison from one testing situation to another could be performed

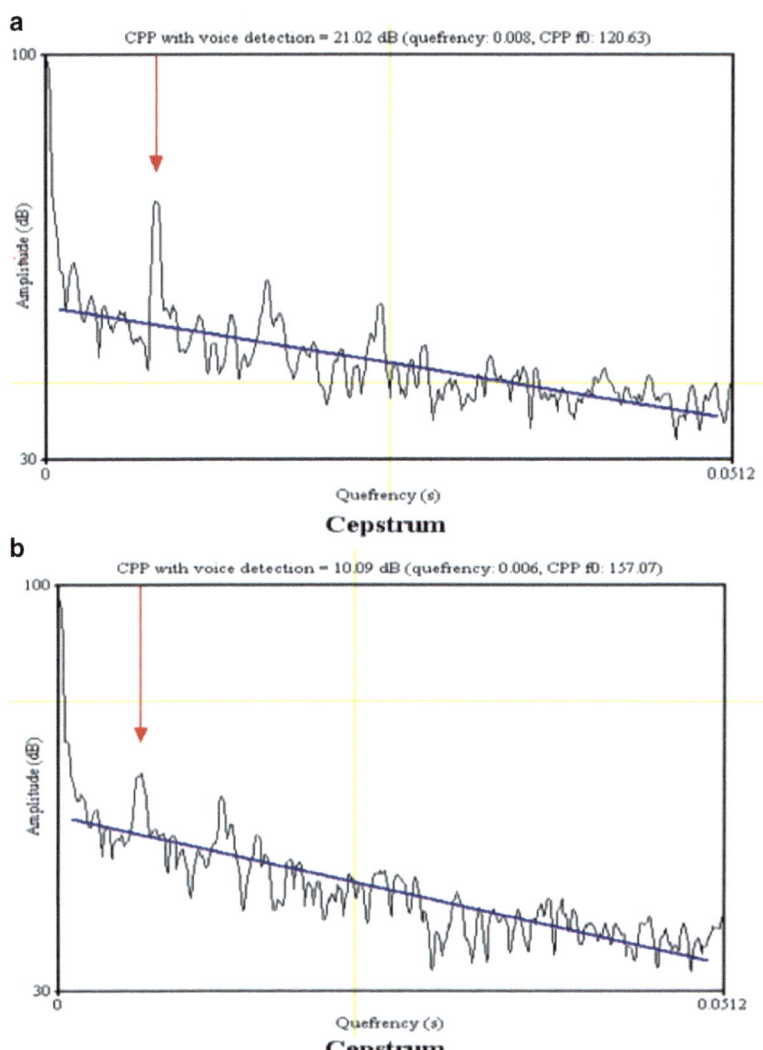

Fig. 10.9 Cepstral measurements. Cepstral representation of normal voice (**a**) and moderately dysphonic voice (**b**)

without having to account for the differences in loudness of phonation, recording level, or microphone distance. These differences could be overcome by adding a linear regression line by the experimenters. Smoothed CPP is another advanced cepstral measure that occurs every 2 ms instead of every 10 ms to reduce artifacts. Brockmann-Bauser et al. [30] advised using the CPP measure of the same vowel for comparison (i.e., the /i/ vowel before management with the /i/ after). They advised detecting age changes in CPP in connected speech better than in vowels. Figure 10.9 illustrates the cepstral representation of a normal voice and moderate dysphonia.

10.2.5 Aerodynamics

Aerodynamics studies the airflow and pressure changes that are produced within the larynx. The commonly used measures include maximum phonation time, mean flow rate, phonation quotient, and subglottal pressure. Kay Elemetric's Phonatory Aerodynamic System (PAS) could be used for the measurement. They point to the hyperfunctional or hypofunctional styles of voice production and to the response to management, despite having a low diagnostic value [31].

Maximum Phonation Time (MPT)

It is the maximum time spent by a person to sustain a vowel produced in a single breath with comfortable loudness and pitch. This is represented in seconds. It measures the glottic efficiency by depicting the ability of the VFs to be efficiently adducted and to vibrate via rapid cycles of opening and closing. The presence of laryngeal pathology will result in reduced MPT as a result of a reduction in glottic efficiency. It is used to evaluate simple respiratory functions and can be performed anywhere without special instruments. It has been found that even obesity affects the MPT. As the body mass index increases, the MPT decreases [32].

Mean Flow Rate (MFR)

It can be measured as individuals maintaining a steady vowel with a balloon valve interrupting their airflow (five times for 250 milliseconds each). MFR is sensitive to changes in glottic configuration and biomechanics. It rises in lesions such as VF polyps [33].

Maximum Flow Declination Rate (MFDR)

This refers to the fastest rate of change in airflow during the closing phase. MFDR is the most negative peak of the differentiated glottal airflow waveform. After this negative peak, the glottal airflow waveform time derivative returns to zero because phonation goes into the closed phase. It is an indirect estimate of the maximum VF closing velocity. It is measured by a flow glottogram. This is related to the relative magnitude of the vocal fold collision forces. This was also related to the vibrational amplitude ratio and vocal tract inertance. It depends on the ratio between the cartilaginous and membranous portions of the VFs, increased amplitude of VF vibration, increased mucosa thickness, increased vocal tract loading, and increased magnitude of the airflow through the glottis. A greater amplitude of vibration results in a greater recoil of the VFs. A higher peak of airflow through the glottis may lead to a quicker return of the VFs to the closed position by virtue of a greater Bernoulli effect. Both situations raise the MFDR. It has been reported to show a positive correlation with increased voice intensity [34].

10.2.6 Voice Range Profile (Phonetogram)

A phonetogram is the plotting of the dynamic range of the voice as a function of F0. It is advised to be used for singing students or professional singers who have complaints in singing, especially with negative stroboscopic findings. It requires patients to produce the maximum variations in F0 at the minimum and maximum intensity levels while producing a certain vowel in ascending and descending pitch glides to represent the voice capacity. Improvements in laryngeal muscle tone and strength, in addition to improved balance among laryngeal muscles and balanced respiratory effort and control, might result in a rise in the vocal capacities [35].

10.2.7 Electroglottography (EGG)

It is a device for measuring the VF contact area during voice production. The signal of EGG waveforms represents variations in the impedance of the vocal tract and the neck tissues produced in response to high-frequency current, reflecting the conductivity between the VFs. It depends on the proximity of the VFs when judging the VF contact area. It has two electrodes, which are placed on each side of a person's thyroid cartilage [36]. The open quotient and closed quotient are the commonly used measures. These quotients could also be evaluated by kymography [15]. The open quotient is the time the VFs are separated from each other, divided by the duration of the whole glottal cycle. The open quotient (OQ) for hypofunctional dysphonia was higher than that for hyperfunctional dysphonia in the anterior and middle, but not posterior, parts of the VF. It was observed to be high in leukoplakia. Dysphonic voices have higher values of OQ than normal voices because of the long open phase intervals. A variation in the open quotient with vocal intensity in speech and singing has been reported [37]. The closed quotient is the ratio between the closed phase and the whole glottal cycle. A low closed quotient was noticed in mutational dysphonia [15].

10.2.8 Inverse Filtering

It represents the glottal waveform by removing the effect of the estimated lip and vocal tract radiations from the output speech waveform. A commonly used measure of inverse filtering is the open quotient. In dysphonia, the open quotient has higher values than in a normal voice because of the long open phase intervals [6]. See also the chapters by Paavo Alku and Ramón Hernandéz Villoria in this book.

10.3 Discussion

Identifying the pathological changes of voice-related biomarkers would help clinicians and researchers determine the possible causes of dysphonia, predict the progress of the disorder, properly manage the problem, and set basis for the future early detection of the disorders participating in developing dysphonia. The clinical history and physical examination for dysphonic patients have only 5% diagnostic accuracy compared to 68% accuracy with the use of initial evaluation by endoscopic laryngoscopy [38]. The measures highlighted by the European laryngologists and phoniatricians in Lechien et al. [3] provided clinical and instrumental tools that could be used in different research and/or clinical facilities in developed and developing countries. This could expand the possibility of validated data, setting hope for unlimited collaboration between health care professionals across the globe, which is one of the goals of the Biomarkers Committee of the Union of European phoniatricians.

10.4 Conclusion

The voice-related biomarkers are variables to serve as monitors of laryngeal pathologies in different health facilities with variable equipment levels. Biomarkers relying on clinicians, patients, or devices provide a wide variety of voice quality assessments and management for the benefit of patients and research. Some voice-related biomarkers could be used to overcome the limitations of others. For example, some biomarkers could not be used in a severe dysphonic voice. Therefore, others were created to overcome this problem. The factors that control the changes in a biomarker help clinicians determine which biomarkers are better to be included in the voice health plans or in the research studies design.

Acknowledgments We would like to thank and express our deepest gratitude to Major General Prof. Dr. Ahmed M. El-Demerdash, Military Medical Academy, Head of the Phoniatrics, Audiology, and Balance Center, Otorhinolaryngology Department, Kobry Elkobba Armed Forces Hospital, Cairo, Egypt, for providing all the stroposcopic figures of the VFs presented in this chapter.

References

1. Califf RM. Biomarker definitions and their applications. Exp Biol Med (Maywood). 2018;243(3):213–21. https://doi.org/10.1177/1535370217750088.
2. Fujiki RB, Thibeault SL. Pediatric voice therapy: how many sessions to discharge? Am J Speech Lang Pathol. 2022;31(6):2663–74. https://doi.org/10.1044/2022_AJSLP-22-00111.
3. Lechien JR, Geneid A, Bohlender JE, Cantarella G, Avellaneda JC, Desuter G, et al. Consensus for voice quality assessment in clinical practice: guidelines of the European Laryngological Society and Union of the European Phoniatricians. Eur Arch Otorhinolaryngol. 2023 Dec;280(12):5459–73. https://doi.org/10.1007/s00405-023-08211-6.
4. Kotby MN. Voice disorders: recent diagnostic advances. Egypt J Otolaryngol. 1986;3(1):69–98.

5. Sujitha PS, Pebbili GK. Cepstral analysis of voice in young adults. J Voice. 2022;36(1):43–9. https://doi.org/10.1016/j.jvoice.2020.03.010.
6. Vinod H, Sharma RK. Glottal wave analysis of dysphonic voice using inverse filtering. In: 2018 Second International Conference on Intelligent Computing and Control Systems (ICICCS). Madurai; 2018. p. 991–4. https://doi.org/10.1109/ICCONS.2018.8663103.
7. El-Adawy A, Ahmed M, Hassan E, Mohammed IR. Modified GRBAS versus Cape-v scale for assessment of voice quality: correlation with acoustic and aerodynamics measurement for Arabic speaking subjects. Sci Med J. 2011;23(4):1–14.
8. Van Stan JH, Mehta DD, Ortiz AJ, Burns JA, Toles LE, Marks KL, Vangel M, Hron T, Zeitels S, Hillman RE. Differences in weeklong ambulatory vocal behavior between female patients with phonotraumatic lesions and matched controls. J Speech Lang Hear Res. 2020;63(2):372–84. https://doi.org/10.1044/2019_JSLHR-19-00065.
9. Heman-Ackah YD, Ivey CM, Alexander R. Options for treatment of a small glottic gap. Laryngoscope Investig Otolaryngol. 2023;8(3):720–9. https://doi.org/10.1002/lio2.1060.
10. Junuzović-Žunić L, Ibrahimagić A, Altumbabić S. Voice characteristics in patients with thyroid disorders. Eurasian J Med. 2019;51(2):101–5. https://doi.org/10.5152/eurasianjmed.2018.18331.
11. Lundy DS, Casiano RR. Compensatory falsetto: effects on vocal quality. J Voice. 1995;9(4):439–42. https://doi.org/10.1016/s0892-1997(05)80207-3.
12. Zhang Z. Mechanics of human voice production and control. J Acoust Soc Am. 2016;140(4):2614. https://doi.org/10.1121/1.4964509.
13. Dichter BK, Breshears JD, Leonard MK, Chang EF. The control of vocal pitch in human laryngeal motor cortex. Cell Press. 2018;174:21–31.e9.
14. Zhang Z. The physical aspects of vocal health. Acoust Today. 2021;17(3):60–8. https://doi.org/10.1121/at.2021.17.3.60.
15. Szkiełkowska A, Krasnodębska P, Miaśkiewicz B, Włodarczyk E, Domeracka-Kolodziej A, Skarżyński H. Mucosal wave measurements in the diagnosis of functional dysphonia. Otolaryngol Pol. 2019;73(6):1–7. https://doi.org/10.5604/01.3001.0013.3215.
16. Andrade DF, Heuer R, Hockstein NE, Castro E, Spiegel JR, Sataloff RT. The frequency of hard glottal attacks in patients with muscle tension dysphonia, unilateral benign masses and bilateral benign masses. J Voice. 2000;14(2):240–6. https://doi.org/10.1016/s0892-1997(00)80032-6.
17. Xu X, Huang X, Tan J, Stevenson H, Zhuang P, Li X. The effects of hard voice onset on objective voice function in patients with laryngopharyngeal reflux. J Voice. 2024;38(5):1256.e9–1256.e15. https://doi.org/10.1016/j.jvoice.2022.02.027.
18. Martinez-Paredes JF, Alfakir R, Thompson CC, Menton SM, Rutt A. Effect of chronic cough on voice measures in patients with dysphonia. J Voice. 2023;37:251–6. https://doi.org/10.1016/j.jvoice.2020.12.025.
19. Rzepakowska A, Sielska-Badurek E, Żurek M, Osuch-Wójcikiewicz E, Niemczyk K. Narrow band imaging for risk stratification of glottic cancer within leukoplakia. Head Neck. 2018;40:2149–54. https://doi.org/10.1002/hed.25201.
20. Dabirmoghaddam P, Aghajanzadeh M, Erfanian R, Aghazadeh K, Sohrabpour S, Firouzifar M, et al. Comparative study of increased supraglottic activity in normal individuals and those with Muscle Tension Dysphonia (MTD). J Voice. 2021;35:554–8. https://doi.org/10.1016/j.jvoice.2019.12.003.
21. Poburka BJ, Patel R. Laryngeal endoscopic imaging: fundamentals and key concepts for rating selected parameters. Perspect ASHA Spec Interest Groups. 2021;6(4):736–42. https://doi.org/10.1044/2021_PERSP-21-00073.
22. Malki KH, Mesallam TA, Farahat M, Bukhari M, Murry T. Validation and cultural modification of Arabic voice handicap index. Eur Arch Otorhinolaryngol. 2010;267(11):1743–51. https://doi.org/10.1007/s00405-010-1296-x.
23. Muslih I, Herawati S, Pawarti DR. Association between voice handicap index and praat voice analysis in patients with benign vocal cord lesion before and after microscopic laryngeal surgery. Indian J Otolaryngol Head Neck Surg. 2019;71(Suppl 1):482–8. https://doi.org/10.1007/s12070-018-1363-y.

24. Akbari E, Seifpanahi S, Ghorbani A, Izadi F, Torabinezhad F. The effects of size and type of vocal fold polyp on some acoustic voice parameters. Iran J Med Sci. 2018;43(2):158–63.
25. Lovato A, De Colle W, Giacomelli L, Piacente A, Righetto L, Marioni G, de Filippis C. Multi-Dimensional Voice Program (MDVP) vs Praat for assessing euphonic subjects: a preliminary study on the gender-discriminating power of acoustic analysis software. J Voice. 2016 Nov;30(6):765.e1–5. https://doi.org/10.1016/j.jvoice.2015.10.012.
26. Brockmann-Bauser M, Bohlender JE, Mehta DD. Acoustic perturbation measures improve with increasing vocal intensity in individuals with and without voice disorders. J Voice. 2018;32(2):162–8. https://doi.org/10.1016/j.jvoice.2017.04.008.
27. Kreiman J, Gerratt BR. Perceptual interaction of the harmonic source and noise in voice. J Acoust Soc Am. 2012;131(1):492–500. https://doi.org/10.1121/1.3665997.
28. Ferrand CT. Harmonics-to-noise ratio: an index of vocal aging. J Voice. 2002;16(4):480–7. https://doi.org/10.1016/s0892-1997(02)00123-6.
29. Watts CR, Awan SN. Use of spectral/cepstral analyses for differentiating normal from hypofunctional voices in sustained vowel and continuous speech contexts. J Speech Lang Hear Res. 2011;54(6):1525–37. https://doi.org/10.1044/1092-4388(2011/10-0209.
30. Brockmann-Bauser M, Van Stan JH, Carvalho Sampaio M, Bohlender JE, Hillman RE, Mehta DD. Effects of vocal intensity and fundamental frequency on Cepstral Peak prominence in patients with voice disorders and vocally healthy controls. J Voice. 2021;35(3):411–7. https://doi.org/10.1016/j.jvoice.2019.11.015.
31. Sheela S. Laryngeal aerodynamic analysis of vocal nodules. J Laryngol Voice. 2013;3(1):10. https://doi.org/10.4103/2230-9748.118705.
32. Al-Yahya SN, Mohamed Akram MHH, Vijaya Kumar K, Mat Amin SNA, Abdul Malik NA, Mohd Zawawi NA, et al. Maximum phonation time normative values among Malaysians and its relation to body mass index. J Voice. 2022 Jul;36(4):457–63. https://doi.org/10.1016/j.jvoice.2020.07.015.
33. Scholp AJ, Hedberg CD, Lamb JR, Hoffman MR, Braden MN, McMurray JS, Jiang JJ. Measurement reliability of laryngeal resistance and mean flow rate in pediatric subjects. J Voice. 2020 Jul;34(4):590–7. https://doi.org/10.1016/j.jvoice.2019.02.005.
34. Titze IR. Theoretical analysis of maximum flow declination rate versus maximum area declination rate in phonation. J Speech Lang Hear Res. 2006;49(2):439–47. https://doi.org/10.1044/1092-4388(2006/034).
35. Am S, Meijer J, Sulter A. Thesis Chapter 9 effects of voice training on phonetograms and maximum phonation times in female speech therapy students. 2018; https://doi.org/10.13140/RG.2.2.12460.10886.
36. Tomaszewska JZ, Georgakis A. Electroglottography in medical diagnostics of vocal tract pathologies: a systematic review. J Voice. 2023;S0892–1997(23):00388–0. https://doi.org/10.1016/j.jvoice.2023.12.004.
37. Bernardoni NH, d'Alessandro C, Doval B, Castellengo M. Glottal open quotient in singing: measurements and correlation with laryngeal mechanisms, vocal intensity, and fundamental frequency. J Acoust Soc Am. 2005;117(3):1417–30. https://doi.org/10.1121/1.1850031ff.
38. Singh S, Roy M, Mathur NN. Role of videostroboscopy and electroglottography during therapeutic intervention in voice disorders. Int J Otorhinolaryngol Clin. 2021;13(3):106–9.

Open Access This chapter is licensed under the terms of the Creative Commons Attribution-NonCommercial-NoDerivatives 4.0 International License (http://creativecommons.org/licenses/by-nc-nd/4.0/), which permits any noncommercial use, sharing, distribution and reproduction in any medium or format, as long as you give appropriate credit to the original author(s) and the source, provide a link to the Creative Commons license and indicate if you modified the licensed material. You do not have permission under this license to share adapted material derived from this chapter or parts of it.

The images or other third party material in this chapter are included in the chapter's Creative Commons license, unless indicated otherwise in a credit line to the material. If material is not included in the chapter's Creative Commons license and your intended use is not permitted by statutory regulation or exceeds the permitted use, you will need to obtain permission directly from the copyright holder.

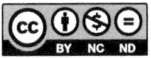

Neurodegenerative Diseases: Aspects of Voice-Related Biomarkers

11

Valentina Camesasca

11.1 Introduction

11.1.1 Neurodegenerative Diseases

Neurodegenerative diseases (NDD) are a vast cluster of neurological disorders with various clinical and pathological manifestations that impact particular subsets of neurons in distinct functional anatomic systems, which debilitate patients' cognitive health and physical abilities, leading to a decline in autonomy and quality of life. The term "neurodegeneration" originated from the word "*neuro*," which indicates nerve cells, and "*degeneration*," which describes a process of losing structure or function in tissues or organs. Thus, talking about neurodegenerative diseases, we are referring to any degenerative disease that predominantly affects neurons. The most prevalent neurodegenerative disease is Parkinson's Disease (PD), which has been described in several chapters. Amyotrophic Lateral Sclerosis (ALS) and Alzheimer's disease (AD) are also prevalent. They affect 15% of the global population and typically have an unexplained beginning and an insidious course. Despite their prevalence, there are few disease-modifying therapies available to prevent or treat neurodegenerative diseases. Therefore, identifying possible voice-related biomarkers to diagnose and monitor these pathologies would be important and useful [1].

11.1.2 Amyotrophic Lateral Sclerosis

Amyotrophic Lateral Sclerosis (ALS) is a neurodegenerative disease characterized by progressive impairment of muscle strength and function due to progressive loss

---

V. Camesasca (✉)
Grande Ospedale Metropolitano Niguarda, Centro Clinico NEMO (NeuroMuscolar Omnicenter), Milano, Italy

of upper (UMNs) and lower (LMNs) motor neurons. This progressive condition may affect a lot or a little of multiple speech subsystems (i.e., respiratory, resonatory/velopharyngeal, voice/phonatory, and articulatory), causing devastating effects on communication [2, 3]. We can identify different clinical phenotypes of Amyotrophic Lateral Sclerosis across individuals: Bulbar, Spinal, and Respiratory. Regardless of the phenotype, over the course of the disease, most of the patients will experience bulbar symptoms affecting speech, feeding, and swallowing. Over 80% of individuals with Amyotrophic Lateral Sclerosis develop dysphonia and dysarthria, primarily a mixed spastic-flaccid subtype resulting from the deterioration of both UMNs and LMNs involved in speech production. Of these, 48% of the patients have dysphonia at onset (mainly bulbar phenotype). Speech impairment may begin up to 3 years prior to the diagnosis of Amyotrophic Lateral Sclerosis, and as the disease progresses over time, there is significant deterioration in speech. Detectable changes in voice quality with the GRBAS test (hoarseness, roughness, strain, and breathiness) or loudness can be identified in patients with Amyotrophic Lateral Sclerosis. Thus, we need to search and develop valid, reliable, and easily implemented measures of dysphonia to early identify bulbar involvement, track bulbar decline over time, and monitor progress during clinical trials [4–6].

11.1.3 Alzheimer's Disease

Alzheimer's disease (AD) is a neurodegenerative disease characterized by memory loss, language dysfunction, and various cognitive disorders, which ultimately leads to patients' loss of independent living ability [7, 8]. With the aging of the world population, this disease will bring a great burden to the families concerned and may cause great social and economic pressure. The number of patients will reach 152 million by 2050. The early stage of Mild Cognitive Impairment (MCI) is a key phase in deciding whether AD can be controlled or not and in stopping or slowing down the disease from developing into dementia in later stages. The definitive diagnosis of AD is made through cerebrospinal fluid analysis, researching $A\beta$ and protein Tau, but it is expensive, painful, and risky. Also, typical radiological modifications in MRI and PET could be useful to diagnose AD. Alternatively, we have several scales and questionnaires (i.e., Montreal Cognitive Assessment (MoCA), Clinical Dementia Rating (CDR), Mini-Mental State Exams (MMSE), and Alzheimer's Disease Assessment Scale Cognitive-Subscale (ADAS-cog)), but they don't achieve sufficiently high accuracy or reliability. Therefore, we have an urgent need to develop a more effective and less risky method to diagnose Alzheimer's Disease [7].

11.2 Perspectives

11.2.1 Voice-Related Biomarkers in Amyotrophic Lateral Sclerosis

The complexity of neurodegenerative diseases, in which multiple speech subsystems may be affected, complicates the direct assessment of single subsystems since each may have a significant confounding effect on the measurement of the others [2, 3]. Voice analysis in Amyotrophic Lateral Sclerosis is also complicated by the variable manifestation of the disease across individuals and within an individual across time. Moreover, the involvement of upper motor neurons (UMNs) and lower motor neurons (LMNs) results in extremely different phonatory disorders, with UMN dysfunction producing spastic dysphonia and LMN dysfunction producing flaccid dysphonia [2]. Therefore, these typical features of ALS may impact auditory-perceptual and cepstral/spectral measures, with consequent limitations in voice evaluation.

Traditional (Perturbation/Noise-Based) Acoustic Measures Among the most commonly used acoustic measures for quantifying dysphonia in Amyotrophic Lateral Sclerosis have been *jitter* (measure of cycle-to-cycle variation in frequency), *shimmer* (measure of cycle-to-cycle variation in amplitude), and *harmonics-to-noise ratio* (HNR) (measure of turbulent noise present in the voice signal). These traditional acoustic measures reflect the amount of involuntary variation (perturbation) in vocal signals. These features can be considered acoustic correlates of perceptual measures of voice; both jitter and shimmer have primarily been associated with perceived roughness and overall voice quality, whereas HNR has been associated with perceived breathiness and roughness. However, the existing literature related to the acoustic characterization of dysphonia in ALS is limited by several methodological factors. The reliability of jitter values may decrease as the severity of dysphonia increases. Furthermore, perturbation analysis is limited to sustained vowels produced at a steady pitch because the characteristics of continuous speech (such as short vowel durations, fundamental frequency variation, pauses, and voiceless consonants) may significantly impact these measures. Therefore, there are many psychometric limitations to traditional acoustic measures [2].

Cepstral/Spectral Measures A growing body of literature has demonstrated the utility of cepstral and spectral approaches (e.g., cepstral peak prominence (CPP), low-high spectral ratio (L/H ratio), and related features) as an alternative to traditional acoustic measures for objectively measuring dysphonia. The advantage of these measures is that they can be extracted from continuous speech and that they may be more reliable across the range of impairment severity than traditional features. *CPP* is higher in voices with strong periodicity and lower in voices characterized by aperiodic noise, and it is correlated with perceptual features of overall dysphonia and breathiness. *CPP SD* reflects the frequency and amplitude variations in normal speech patterns. The *L/H ratio* permits differentiation of normal from dysphonic voices and correlates with perceptual features of overall dysphonia and breathiness. *L/H ratio SD* reflects variability across the duration of a voice sample: a higher value corresponds to better laryngeal support for dynamic adjustments of the larynx, particularly in continuous speech. When using cepstral/spectral values, it is important to consider that the nature of the speech stimulus can affect these measures. CPP values differ significantly when measured during a sustained vowel or during a continuous speech from the same speaker. Moreover, different sentences included in the protocol for CAPE-V [2] have different levels of correlation, and none of those correlations is as strong as the correlation with a sustained vowel. Therefore, the use of a variety of stimuli during clinical voice assessment is recommended to overcome the effects of glottal and supraglottal differences on acoustic measurements [2].

Sustained Vowel Task Jitter, shimmer, and HNR are robust acoustic measures of dysphonia, and they strongly correlate with auditory-perceptual features of vocal dysfunction: roughness, breathiness, strain, and overall dysphonia severity. Jitter and shimmer are especially related to roughness and breathiness, and they correlate with the onset of laryngeal weakness and decreased laryngeal control. Considering the sustained vowel task, patients with Amyotrophic Lateral Sclerosis also show an increased HNR, which reflects turbulent noise due to incomplete glottal closure, and an increased fundamental frequency (F0), which is due to the dysfunction of intrinsic laryngeal muscles. Moreover, patients with ALS typically have a decreased maximum phonation time (MPT), which is due to the reduced control system of vocal fold movement and progressive weakness of respiratory support for voice production. Therefore, traditional acoustic measures may be useful to discriminate bulbar involvement. Voice analysis of patients with ALS demonstrates a significant correlation between cepstral/spectral acoustic features using sustained vowel tasks and perceptual ratings. CPP strongly correlates with breathiness, CSID correlates with both strain and overall dysphonia severity, and L/H ratio SD correlates with roughness, strain, and overall dysphonia severity. These measures better discriminate between dysphonic and non-dysphonic voices and perform well even with low levels of dysphonia [2, 3].

Continuous Speech During continuous speech, cepstral measures may be affected by fluctuations in several laryngeal and articulatory factors, including vocal intensity, fundamental frequency, sound pressure level, syllable stress, vowel context, and vowel type. However, continuous speech is more representative of habitual voice use patterns containing pitch and loudness variations, which serve as important perceptual indicators of vocal dysfunction. Cepstral/spectral measures are strongly associated with perceptual features: CPP with strain, CPP SD with breathiness, and L/H ratio with breathiness, strain, and overall dysphonia. CPP SD is also sensitive to features of continuous speech that impact the variability in the voice signal's periodicity, such as changes in the vowel spectrum and changes in the frequency spectrum due to intonation patterns [2]. We need to consider that in patients with ALS, acoustic assessment of continuous speech is also complicated by various factors related to dysarthric speech and that the deterioration of the resonatory (i.e., velopharyngeal function) and phonatory subsystems frequently occurs prior to articulatory subsystem decline [2]. Therefore, particular characteristics of motor speech disorders (e.g., reduced articulation rate, reduced vowel space, and increased frequency and length of pausing) may confound cepstral/spectral acoustic measures when applied to patients with complex neurodegenerative diseases. Additionally, hypernasality and mixed spastic-flaccid dysarthria with reduced intelligibility associated with ALS may eliminate the straightforward correlation among individuals with complex neurodegenerative diseases, with consequent inescapable bias in acoustic measures.

Hypernasality Hypernasality is a distinctive perceptual feature of speech resonance caused by velopharyngeal dysfunction and is typical of many neurodegenerative diseases, especially ALS. Acoustically, hypernasality is characterized by a reduction in the amplitude of the first formant (F1), the presence of an extra pole (or nasal formant) between the first and second formants, shifting of the center of the low-frequency spectral prominence, an increased amplitude of the bands between F1 and F2, and a decreased amplitude in the F2 region [4]. Because hypernasality is an excessive nasal resonance that occurs on vowels and voiced consonants, several acoustic indices based on voice spectral analysis may correlate with the perceptual evaluation of this specific feature: difference between the amplitude of F1 and the amplitude of the extra peak (A–P1), where P1 is located between F1 and F2; difference between the amplitude of F1 and the amplitude of the first nasal peak P0, which, compared to P1, is lower in peak frequency and located below the F1; voice low tone (below 600 Hz) to high tone (above 600 Hz) spectral ratio; and the one-third octave spectral analysis [4].

Cepstral/spectral measures better reflect the underlying pathophysiology of hypernasality and demonstrate stronger associations with perceptual evaluations of voice quality. CPP and L/H ratio may reflect not only the periodicity of vocal fold vibration but also the filtering effects and resonant function of the vocal tract. However, concurrent impairments in the velopharyngeal mechanism and voice subsystem may confound the effects on spectral energy, causing misunderstandings. Indeed, voice impairments are often characterized by increased energy (noise) at higher frequencies, yielding lower L/H spectral ratio values than in unimpaired speakers. In contrast, hypernasality causes a reduced amplitude of spectral energy at higher frequencies, potentially resulting in a higher L/H spectral ratio [4].

One-third octave analysis using the frequency band centered at 1600 Hz better differentiates asymptomatic patients, patients with predominant hypernasality, and patients with predominant voice impairment. Therefore, it yields the power to be used as an early indicator in neurodegenerative diseases. A one-third octave analysis is able to capture subsystem-specific alterations in distinct frequency bands: below the band centered at 1600 Hz, it captures pronounced impairment in the resonance subsystem (velopharyngeal mechanism), centered at 1600 Hz and above; instead, it captures impaired voice quality as well as impairment in voice and resonance subsystems [4].

CPP is also a sensitive acoustic measure, but it varies depending on the speech task/stimuli, vocal tract configuration, and intensity. Nasalized vowels are associated with reduced CPP, while nasal sentences (with nasal consonants) are characterized by increased CPP. It decreases in patients with predominantly voice impairment, while it increases in patients with predominant hypernasality, which may explain the lack of distinction between patients with hypernasality and voice impairment and asymptomatic patients (reduced CPP due to voice impairment may be canceled out by an increase due to hypernasality) [4]. Hypernasality facilitates phonation and improves the synchronized harmonic organization of voice; it decreases the open quotient of the vibratory cycle by inducing increased muscular adductor forces of vocal folds, independent of intensity or vocal loudness. Moreover, the presence of strong low-frequency spectral energy in nasal resonance may lead to increased CPP. After all, patients with ALS commonly show impairments in all speech subsystems, including articulatory and respiratory subsystems, which may influence CPP measures.

Some authors demonstrated the correlations of the *L/H spectral ratio* with hypernasality rating at a specific cutoff frequency (i.e., 600 Hz), while others did not find such associations [4]. Hypernasality causes increased spectral energy (amplitude) of the frequency bands between F1 and F2 and reduced amplitude around 2500 Hz. Voice impairment, instead, is often characterized by increased energy (noise) at higher frequencies, yielding lower L/H spectral ratio values than unimpaired speakers. Therefore, several controversies exist regarding the use of these acoustic measures in neurodegenerative diseases.

To sum up, one-third of octave analyses and the CPP measure have high classification accuracy for identifying asymptomatic patients from those with hypernasality (velopharyngeal impairment). CPP yields higher predictive power for differentiating asymptomatic people from those with perceived voice impairment, while one-third octave analyses have greater accuracy for distinguishing asymptomatic patients from those with hypernasality and voice impairment [2–4]. Especially, the one-third octave frequency band centered at 1600 Hz may be a strong and reliable acoustic biomarker in neurodegenerative diseases with the potential to distinguish asymptomatic people from patients with hypernasality, voice, and mixed hypernasality and voice impairment.

Voice Onset Time (VOT) VOT is a measure of the temporal difference between an articulatory stop release and the onset of vocal fold vibrations. It is an index frequently used to describe the coordination between the articulatory and laryngeal systems during speech, and it is an important acoustic cue for the voiced–voiceless distinction [5]. Patients in the late stage of Amyotrophic Lateral Sclerosis have significantly longer lead VOT values, whereas there are no differences in VOT between early-stage ALS and healthy people. Patients with more severe ALS showed a greater occurrence of voicing leads and longer voicing leads. Voicing precedes articulatory onset with disease progression in the production of bilabial stops, which suggests that the relative timing of coordination between the supralaryngeal structures and phonatory system is affected in the late stage of ALS [5]. There is a direct relationship between the respiratory and phonatory subsystems, probably because they share the same neural circuitry, but impaired respiration showed more impact on voicing than on articulation.

The respiratory subsystem, particularly low lung volume, is associated with a shortened VOT. In fact, for the production of stops, the difference between intraoral pressure and subglottal pressure determines when voicing occurs. In ALS patients, during the production of the voiced word-initial stops, glottal pulsing precedes the stop release, suggesting that the laryngeal system is activated prior to the build-up of intraoral pressure for the stop. Three possible adjustments to the articulatory-laryngeal subsystems could occur while maintaining or initiating phonation during the closure in voiced stops: a passive supraglottal expansion; an active enlargement of the cavity by adjustments like larynx lowering, tongue root advancement, and tongue body lowering; and nasal airflow through an incomplete velopharyngeal closure.

Patients with late-stage ALS have a longer negative (lead) VOT, which may be due to impaired lip and jaw movements and supraglottal leakage from weakness in velopharyngeal closure. In fact, during the production of bilabial stop consonants, lips move at a high velocity at the onset of oral closure, resulting in tissue compression and an airtight seal for intraoral pressure buildup. In healthy people, there are adjustments that enable flexible control using either a voicing lead or a short-lag voicing mode. Findings of reduced flexible mode of voicing (lead vs. short lag) and inverse correlation between VOT and intelligible speaking rate may be indicative of neurodegenerative changes that occur with disease severity in ALS. Changes in VOT with speech decline in patients with ALS could be considered as a progressive loss of phonetic features, such as voiced-voiceless contrast and oral versus nasal contrasts in later stages of the disease. The coordination between the articulatory and phonatory speech subsystems may also be influenced by individual differences in neural degeneration localization: different phenotypes (bulbar, spinal, and respiratory) and different prevalence in late-stage ALS (bulbar symptomatic—high speech function vs. low speech function).

To sum up, patients in late-stage ALS have a longer lead VOT than patients with early-stage ALS and healthy people. VOT duration increases with increasing severity of speech symptoms in patients with ALS. VOT reflects impaired temporal coordination between the laryngeal and supralaryngeal structures. Longer lead VOT in late-stage ALS reflects neurodegenerative changes due to disease progression. Voicing leads occur predominantly in late-stage ALS, suggesting that laryngeal and articulatory coordination changes with disease progression [5].

Machine Learning Voice Analysis New technologies, Machine Learning and Artificial Intelligence, may be extremely useful to perform voice analysis in neurodegenerative diseases. Tena et al., in their study, used machine learning voice analysis to demonstrate that the performance of the automated diagnosis of bulbar involvement may be superior to human diagnosis. With this technology, a total of 15 acoustic features were extracted [6]: jitter(absolute), jitter(relative), jitter(rap), jitter(ppq5), shimmer(relative), shimmer(dB), shimmer(apq3), shimmer(apq5), shimmer(apq11), pitch(mean), pitch(SD), pitch(min), pitch(max), HNR(mean), and HNR(SD). They demonstrated that acoustic analysis of vowels elicited from patients with ALS may be used for early detection of bulbar involvement and that this could be done automatically using supervised classification models. The authors have also shown that there was better performance by applying principal component analysis (PCA) previously to the obtained features and that bulbar involvement can be detected using automatic tools before it becomes perceptible to human hearing. The results point to the importance of obtaining objective measures to allow an early and more accurate diagnosis, given that humans may often misdiagnose this deficiency [6].

11.2.2 Voice-Related Biomarkers in Alzheimer's Disease

Subtle changes in voice and language can be observed years before the appearance of prodromal symptoms of Alzheimer's disease: alterations in verbal fluency, reflected by the patient's hesitation to speak and slow speech rate; word-finding difficulties, leading to circumlocution and frequent use of filler sounds (e.g., uh, and um); semantic errors, indefinite terms, revision, repetitions, and neologisms; lexical and grammatical simplification; loss of semantic abilities in general; discourse characterized by reduced coherence, with implausible and irrelevant details; and alterations perceived in prosodic features (pitch variation and modulation and speech rhythm) [7, 8]. Therefore, voice features have the potential to become simple and noninvasive biomarkers for the early diagnosis of AD and, more generally, conditions associated with dementia.

Formants F1—F2—F3 and Voice Onset Time (VOT) Patients with Alzheimer's disease show a different inclination in vowel space configurations, with significant differences, especially in F3 of /u/. F3 of the vowel /u/ is usually related to lip rounding. The production of /u/ requires higher spatiotemporal constraints, and its production necessitates two simultaneous constrictions, a bilabial and a tongue-dorsum, in the velar region [7]. Patients with AD also showed higher VOT values, particularly for consonant the /t/. The consonant /t/ is likely to be the most affected because it requires high gestural celerity, together with a very precise tongue-tip contact for occlusion [7].

Automatic Voice Analyzer and Automatic Speech Recognition Software The Automatic Voice Analyzer is able to automatically analyze temporal and acoustic voice markers to flag the onset of preclinical Alzheimer's disease. The automatic Speech Recognition Software is able to acoustically distinguish early stages of AD using prosodic cues related to pitch (e.g., rate of vocal fold vibration during voiced segments of speech), voicing (e.g., percentage of speech produced utilizing vocal folds such as vowel sounds as opposed to unvoiced harsher sounds usually associated with consonants), and speaking rate and formant energy (e.g., spectral shape of energy in voiced sounds) [8]. Therefore, these new technological systems may be useful to find voice-related biomarkers in patients with AD.

Machine Learning and Deep Learning-Based Speech Analysis Some studies in which new technologies such as Machine Learning and Deep Learning are used show promising results regarding possible voice-related biomarkers in Alzheimer's disease. It has been shown that the Lexical-Semantic Index is sensitive to amyloid positivity, it has a higher diagnostic accuracy, and it is associated with disease progression. Acoustic scores are sensitive to cognitive status and are more sensitive to amyloid status in prodromal versus preclinical AD [9, 10]. These preliminary findings suggest that digital voice biomarkers might not only be able to detect cognitive impairment using brief audio recordings but also to distinguish AD clinical status and disease progression.

11.3 Discussion

Neurodegenerative diseases are a vast cluster of neurological disorders with various clinical and pathological manifestations that impair patients' cognitive health and physical abilities, leading to a decline in their autonomy and quality of life. They affect 15% of the global population, and they typically have an unexplained beginning and an insidious course. The most prevalent neurodegenerative diseases are Parkinson's disease (PD), Amyotrophic Lateral Sclerosis (ALS), and Alzheimer's disease (AD). Amyotrophic Lateral Sclerosis is characterized by progressive impairment of muscle strength and function due to progressive loss of upper and lower motor neurons. This progressive condition affects multiple speech subsystems (respiratory, resonatory/velopharyngeal, voice/phonatory, and articulatory), causing devastating effects on communication. Over 80% of individuals with ALS develop dysphonia and dysarthria, and 48% of patients present dysphonia at onset. Speech impairment may begin up to 3 years prior to diagnosis of Amyotrophic Lateral Sclerosis, and as the disease progresses over time, there is significant deterioration in speech.

However, the complexity of the disease, in which multiple speech subsystems may be affected, complicates the direct assessment of single subsystems since each may have a significant confounding effect on the measurement of the others. Both traditional (perturbation/noise-based) and cepstral/spectral acoustic measures may be useful for detecting changes in voice quality in patients with ALS. Jitter, shimmer, and harmonics-to-noise ratio are features that reflect the amount of involuntary variation (perturbation) in the vocal signal, and they can be considered acoustic correlates of the perceptual measures of voice.

CPP and L/H ratio are alternative acoustic measures for objectively detecting voice impairment, but they offer the advantage of being extracted from continuous speech and being more reliable across the range of impairment severity than traditional features. It is important to consider that cepstral/spectral measures can be affected by the nature of the speech stimulus (sustained vowel task or continuous speech). Indeed, the specific characteristics of motor speech disorders (e.g., reduced articulation rate, reduced vowel space, and increased frequency and length of pausing), hypernasality, and mixed spastic-flaccid dysarthria with reduced intelligibility typical of ALS may confound acoustic measures with consequent inescapable bias in acoustic measures.

Hypernasality is a specific perceptual feature of speech resonance due to velopharyngeal dysfunction. It is typical of many neurodegenerative diseases, especially ALS, and is associated with specific acoustic modifications regarding formants, cepstral/spectral measures, and one-third octave analysis. Voice Onset Time (VOT) is another important feature that may be impaired in NDD. This is a measure of the temporal difference between articulatory stop release and the onset of vocal-fold vibrations. It is frequently used to describe the coordination between the articulatory and laryngeal systems during speech, and it is an important acoustic cue for the voiced–voiceless distinction. Alzheimer's disease is characterized by memory loss, language dysfunction, and various cognitive disorders, which ultimately lead to patients' loss of independent living ability.

With the aging of the world population, this disease will bring a great burden to the families concerned and may cause great social and economic pressure. The early-stage Mild Cognitive Impairment (MCI) test is a key phase in deciding whether AD can be controlled or not and in stopping or slowing down the disease from developing into dementia in later stages. Subtle changes in voice and language can be observed years before the appearance of the prodromal symptoms of Alzheimer's disease. Therefore, voice features have the potential to become simple and noninvasive biomarkers for the early diagnosis of AD and, more generally, conditions associated with dementia. Patients with AD show an inclination in vowel space configurations, with significant differences in formants and higher VOT values. New technologies, such as Artificial Intelligence, Machine Learning, and Deep Learning, used in the Automatic Voice Analyzer and the Speech Recognition Software, may be extremely useful in performing voice analysis in neurodegenerative diseases. Different studies have demonstrated that they may be superior to humans in identifying subtle preclinical voice impairment [8–10].

11.4 Conclusion

Neurodegenerative diseases are relatively common diseases that typically have an unexplained beginning and an insidious course. Despite their prevalence, there are few disease-modifying therapies available to prevent or treat them. Therefore, identifying possible voice-related biomarkers to diagnose and monitor these pathologies would be highly important and useful. There are several studies that have shown promising results regarding possible voice-related digital biomarkers in NDD [4, 10], but we need large clinical trials to confirm them.

References

1. Cheslow L, Snook AE, Waldman SA. Biomarkers for managing neurodegenerative diseases. Biomolecules. 2024;14(4):398. https://doi.org/10.3390/biom14040398.
2. Maffei MF, Green JR, Murton O, Yunusova Y, Rowe HP, Wehbe F, et al. Acoustic measures of dysphonia in amyotrophic lateral sclerosis. J Speech Lang Hear Res. 2023;66(3):872–87. https://doi.org/10.1044/2022_JSLHR-22-00363.
3. Chiaramonte R, Bonfiglio M. Acoustic analysis of voice in bulbar amyotrophic lateral sclerosis: a systematic review and meta-analysis of studies. Logoped Phoniatr Vocol. 2020 Dec;45(4):151–63. https://doi.org/10.1080/14015439.2019.1687748.
4. Eshghi M, Connaghan KP, Gutz SE, Berry JD, Yunusova Y, Green JR. Co-occurrence of hypernasality and voice impairment in amyotrophic lateral sclerosis: acoustic quantification. J Speech Lang Hear Res. 2021;64(12):4772–83. https://doi.org/10.1044/2021_JSLHR-21-00123.
5. Thomas A, Teplansky KJ, Wisler A, Heitzman D, Austin S, Wang J. Voice onset time in early- and late-stage amyotrophic lateral sclerosis. J Speech Lang Hear Res. 2022;65(7):2586–93. https://doi.org/10.1044/2022_JSLHR-21-00632.
6. Tena A, Claria F, Solsona F, Meister E, Povedano M. Detection of bulbar involvement in patients with amyotrophic lateral sclerosis by machine learning voice analysis: diagnostic decision support development study. JMIR Med Inform. 2021;9(3):e21331. https://doi.org/10.2196/21331.
7. Xiu N, Vaxelaire B, Li L, Ling Z, Xu X, Huang L, Sun B, Huang L, Sock R. A study on voice measures in patients with Alzheimer's disease. J Voice. 2025 Jan;39(1):286.e13–24. https://doi.org/10.1016/j.jvoice.2022.08.010.
8. Martínez-Sánchez F, Meilán JJG, Carro J, Ivanova O. A prototype for the voice analysis diagnosis of Alzheimer's disease. J Alzheimer's Dis. 2018;64(2):473–81. https://doi.org/10.3233/JAD-180037.
9. Yang Q, Li X, Ding X, Xu F, Ling Z. Deep learning-based speech analysis for Alzheimer's disease detection: a literature review. Alzheimer's Res Ther. 2022;14(1) https://doi.org/10.1186/s13195-022-01131-3.
10. Hajjar I, Okafor M, Choi JD, Moore E 2nd, Abrol A, Calhoun VD, Goldstein FC. Development of digital voice biomarkers and associations with cognition, cerebrospinal biomarkers, and neural representation in early Alzheimer's disease. Alzheimers Dement (Amst). 2023;15(1):e12393. https://doi.org/10.1002/dad2.12393.

Open Access This chapter is licensed under the terms of the Creative Commons Attribution-NonCommercial-NoDerivatives 4.0 International License (http://creativecommons.org/licenses/by-nc-nd/4.0/), which permits any noncommercial use, sharing, distribution and reproduction in any medium or format, as long as you give appropriate credit to the original author(s) and the source, provide a link to the Creative Commons license and indicate if you modified the licensed material. You do not have permission under this license to share adapted material derived from this chapter or parts of it.

The images or other third party material in this chapter are included in the chapter's Creative Commons license, unless indicated otherwise in a credit line to the material. If material is not included in the chapter's Creative Commons license and your intended use is not permitted by statutory regulation or exceeds the permitted use, you will need to obtain permission directly from the copyright holder.

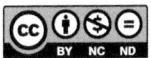

Genetics and the Application of Voice-Related Biomarkers

12

Mette Pedersen and Neveen Hassan Nashaat

12.1 Introduction

In the book Phoniatrics One [1], one chapter focuses on the relationship between voice, vocal folds, and genetic disorders. Numerous studies have been conducted on genetic disorders and their treatment [2, 3]. We have been interested in looking at the use of voice-related biomarkers in the area of genetic disorders, especially since we, as experts, were asked to evaluate a breakthrough article where a genetic link to the fundamental frequency of the voice was identified (Washington's post) [4]. In an Icelandic article, a comparison was made between the acoustical voice parameters of pitch and the genomic analysis of 12,901 Islanders. A connection was found among the ABCC9 genetic variants.

A consensus paper by the Union of European Phoniatricians (UEP) and the European Laryngology Society (ELS) [5] provides an overview of updated recommendations for voice measurements in clinical practice. As for the Icelandic study, it can be questioned whether a small number of acoustic parameters alone can be used in such a large genetic comparison situation (80 parameters from the free PRAAT software against the genomes of the 12,901 Islanders).

The UEP committee of voice-related biomarkers suggests, as a minimum for non-invasive evaluation: patient complaints, Voice Handicap Index (VHI); listener's evaluations GRBAS test; acoustic parameters—fundamental frequency (F0), jitter, shimmer, harmonics to noise (HNR); airflow, and maximum phonation time (MPT).

M. Pedersen (✉)
The Medical Center, Copenhagen, Denmark
e-mail: M.f.pedersen@dadlnet.dk

N. H. Nashaat
Research on Children with Special Needs Department, Medical Research and Clinical Studies Institute, National Research Centre, Cairo, Egypt

© The Author(s) 2026
M. Pedersen et al. (eds.), *Voice-related Biomarkers*,
https://doi.org/10.1007/978-3-032-03134-1_12

This correlates with the UEP/ELS consensus paper 2023 [5]. This aspect indicates that a combined score will be possible in the future based on computer foundation models.

12.2 Perspectives

To investigate the presence of the UEP Voice-Related Biomarkers Committee's suggestions in the literature of genetics, a collaboration was undertaken with the Royal Society of Medicine (RSM) library in the UK. The aim was to identify which measures are employed for both normal and pathological voices in genetic studies. This area is new, and many authors, especially those in genetic neurology, have commented that their study is the first on voice-related measures. Consequently, we decided to analyze the literature from the past 5 years up to October 18, 2024. In Table 12.1, the search setup is presented. The results of the library search can be received at the request of the first author.

The search for measures of normal voices in genetic connections gave few results, especially regarding F0 [6]. This study confirms the breakthrough made by Gisladottir et al. [4]. It is now widely recognized that voices have a genetic basis, particularly from a developmental perspective [7]. A measurable genetic difference was found between normal singers and non-singers [8, 9]. The relation to FOXP2 genes for auditory feedback is another aspect [10]. It brings forward the viewpoint that genes are related to lower and higher brain activity and voice [10]. In the literature on genetics and laryngeal cancer heterogeneity, voice-related biomarkers were not utilized (yet) [11].

Tables 12.2 and 12.3 summarize the genetic studies on pathology identified in the search that include voice measurements. These studies are described concerning the previously outlined voice-related biomarkers: VHI, GRBAS test, acoustic parameters such as F0, jitter, shimmer, HNR (or NHR), and MPT. These

Table 12.1 Library search. Presents the setup for the search at the Royal Society of Medicine Library, UK, including limits

Search 1
GENETIC studies that include MEASUREMENT of the normal voice:
Pitch and vowel acoustics
Other voice measures
Vocal fold measures
Search 2
Focus on the GENETIC studies that include pathological voice MEASUREMENTS:
Pitch and vowel acoustics
Other voice measures
Vocal fold measures
Limits for both searches
Last 5 years (2019–2024)
All languages
Human studies only
All studies and publication types

Table 12.2 Overview of papers on genetic disorders that include voice analysis up to 2024. Shows the papers that include voice analysis. There are massive differences between the topics, so it has not been possible to order the papers referring to genetic variance

2024
Saft C, et al. Speech biomarkers in Huntington's disease: A longitudinal follow-up study in Premanifest mutation carriers.
Kao TH et al., Oral Diadochokinetic markers of X-linked dystonia-parkinsonism
2023
Cala F, Artificial intelligence procedure for the screening of genetic syndromes based on voice characteristics
O'Brien ARW et al., Prevalence of voice and swallow problems in individuals living with sickle cell disease
Semmler, M et al., Influence of reduced saliva production on phonation in patients with ectodermal dysplasia
Pelka F et al., Mechanical parameters based on high-speed Videoendoscopy of the vocal folds in patients with ectodermal dysplasia
Frasseneti I et al., Quantitative acoustical analysis of genetic syndromes in the number listing task. Biomedical signal processing and control
Friedman L et al., Atypical vocal quality in women with the FMR1 Premutation: An indicator of impaired sensorimotor control
Jacinto-Scudeiro LA et al., Dysarthria in hereditary spastic paraplegia type 4
2022
Riad R et al., Predicting clinical scores in Huntington's disease: A lightweight speech test
Cordella C et al., Acoustic and kinematic assessment of motor speech impairment in patients with suspected four-repeat Tauopathies
Hseu AF et al., Laryngeal pathologies in dysphonic children with Down syndrome,
Singh R, Connecting human voice profiling to genomics: A predictive algorithm for linking speech phenotypes to genetic microdeletion syndromes
Andrade BMR et al., Impact of Semioccluded vocal tract exercises and choral singing on quality of life in subjects with congenital GH deficiency
Sacconi S et al., Facial and vocal recognition as a decision support tool for neuromuscular diseases: The FACENMD project
2021
Lowell S.Y et al., Clinical features of essential voice tremor and associations with tremor severity and response to Octanoic acid treatment
Kosztyła-Hojna B et al., Phoniatric, audiological, Orodental, and speech problems in a boy with cardio-Facio-cutaneous syndrome type 3 (CFC 3) due to a pathogenic variant in MAP2K1—Case study
Neves PCR et al., Perfil vocal de Indivíduos 46, XX com Hiperplasia adrenal Congênita
Hidalgo-De la Guía I et al., Acoustic analysis of phonation in children with smith–Magenis syndrome.
Hidalgo-De la Guía et al., Specificities of phonation biomechanics in down syndrome children, biomedical signal processing and control
2020
Song SA. et al., Progressive decline in voice and voice-related quality of life in X-linked dystonia parkinsonism

(continued)

Table 12.2 (continued)

Krishnamurthy R et al., Aerodynamic and acoustic characteristics of voice in children with down syndrome-A systematic review
Moya-Mendez ME et al., Auditory-perceptual voice and speech evaluation in ATP1A3 positive patients
Carraro L et al., Phenotypic characterization of a cohort of patients affected by laryngeal dystonia: A monocentric study
Sobuś et al., Humoral influence of repeated lineage-negative stem/progenitor cell administration on articulatory functions in ALS patients
2019
Pebbili GK et al., Laryngeal aerodynamic analysis of glottal Valving in children with Down syndrome
Bartier S et al., Pharyngo-laryngeal involvement in systemic amyloidosis with cardiac involvement: A prospective observational study.
Ali L et al., Automated detection of Parkinson's disease based on multiple types of sustained phonations using linear discriminant analysis and genetically optimized neural network
Kleim K et al., Objective evaluation criteria for diagnosis of spasmodic dysphonia
Spencer KA et al., Dysarthria profiles in adults with hereditary ataxia
Khodadoust M et al., Speech difficulties in Joubert syndrome
Sebastián-Lázaro D et al., Voz y Habla de los Niños con Síndrome de Deleción de 22q11
Nevler N et al., Validated automatic speech biomarkers in primary progressive aphasia
2018
Ebert B et al., Congenital and iatrogenic laryngeal and vocal abnormalities in patients with 22q11
Jackowska J et al., Thyroplasty in unilateral vocal fold paresis with coexisting hereditary hemorrhagic telangiectasia: A case report
Vogel AP et al., Coordination and timing deficits in speech and swallowing in autosomal recessive spastic ataxia of Charlevoix–Saguenay
Konstantopoulos K et al., Quantification of Dysarthrophonia in a Cypriot family with autosomal recessive hereditary spastic paraplegia associated with a homozygous SPG11 mutation
Szklanny K et al., Voice alterations in patients with Morquio A syndrome
Demopoulos, C et al., Abnormal speech motor control in individuals with 16p11
2017
Vogel AP et al., Voice in Friedreich ataxia
Hidalgo I. et al., Biomechanical description of phonation in children affected by Williams syndrome
Vogel AP et al., Speech and swallowing abnormalities in adults with POLG-associated ataxia (POLG-A), mitochondrion
Poujois A et al., Dystonic dysarthria in Wilson disease: Efficacy of zolpidem. Frontiers in neurology
Hintze JM et al., Spasmodic dysphonia: A review. Part 1: Pathogenic factors.
Balasubramaniam RK et al., Voice mutation during adolescence in Mangalore, India: Implications for the assessment and management of mutational voice disorders
Turner SJ et al., Dysarthria and broader motor speech deficits in Dravet syndrome
Wolf AE et al., Phonoarticulation in spinocerebellar ataxia type 3
Montazeri M et al., Voice acoustic and perceptual features in lipoid Proteinosis: A report of two cases

Table 12.3 Papers using one voice-related biomarker. Shows that the fundamental frequency F0 is most often used [61]

VHI:	6
GRBAS:	10
F0:	20
Jitter, shimmer:	8
HNR/NHR:	6
MPT:	6
Machine learning:	5

measures are utilized in the papers, but typically, only one is addressed in each specific study. The overview in Table 12.2 is based on references 12–59, where full information can be found. In the table, we have written the titles to recognize the disorders. Contrary to our expectations, the application of machine learning is less prevalent. The papers related to this topic are compiled in the table. A notable limitation of the literature is the general lack of randomized prospective documentation.

In genetic disorders, F0 is the most commonly used measure (20 cases), in many cases with a standard division and range. As presented in Table 12.3, the other voice-related measures recommended by the UEP committee are also found with VHI 6, GRBAS 10, jitter, shimmer 8, HNR/NHR 6, MPT 6, and machine learning 5 cases. Spectrography is the focus of some papers, as well as cepstrum measures. The overviews in Tables 12.2 and 12.3 underline that the authors used the measures suggested by the UEP committee on voice-related biomarkers. It is seen that not only the mean F0 but also the standard deviation and range of F0 should be included as part of the voice-related biomarkers. The method during the years has become more and more advanced, and only a few use biomarkers as documentation for treatment. Differentiating between the various disorders in groups was too challenging due to the insufficiently detailed descriptions of the conditions in many cases and the extensive variability in genetic structures.

The devices used for measuring various parameters are not always well documented or clearly described.

A future parallel can be drawn with audiometry, where the equipment used for measurements is standardized (e.g., CE in Europe). Unfortunately, this level of standardization has not yet been achieved for devices used in voice measurements.

12.3 Discussion

It is possible to combine analyzing voice parameters from a biomarker's aspect with a standard genomic test (Olink Proteomics AB). As demonstrated in Tables 12.2 and 12.3, voice-related biomarkers are utilized in many genetic disorders; however, they have not been systematically applied, especially to evaluate treatment effects.

The combined measures of several voice-related biomarkers, as suggested by the UEP voice-related biomarkers committee, will be a great opportunity for refining diagnostics and therapeutic procedures in genetic disorders and for providing better aspects of prognoses. As shown in an earlier section, computer power can be used to solve large amounts of data. Computational power can be leveraged to explore additional features and applications for the treatment of genetic disorders, particularly those related to glottic closure, as discussed in other chapters of this book. Nevertheless, voice-related biomarkers serve as fundamental measures for tailoring individual treatment approaches for genetic disorders.

There is a great variability of articles on genetic disorders involving voice, and the voice-related biomarkers seem to be functioning individually. A combination of several aspects of voice, as presented, would be much more sufficient. Future factors may include lower and higher brain function differences based on larger numbers of clients using machine learning. This combination may also give a better genetic understanding of, e.g., talented people. In gene-related cancer diagnostics, voice-related biomarkers could be valuable in conducting randomized controlled trials for diagnosis, treatment, and prognosis.

Direct endoscopy, including high-speed films, is not discussed in this paper, as it is an invasive procedure, but in the future, biomarkers based on Optical Coherence Tomography can be defined. They illustrate the function and tissue of the vocal folds.

12.4 Conclusion

With the help of RSM librarians, we examined papers on genetics for the suggested non-invasive biomarkers during the last 5 years (VHI, the GRBAS test, acoustic measures of F0, jitter, shimmer, HNR, and MPT). They are used, but nearly always only one of them at a time, and F0 at the most. The authors often commented that the measurement of a voice-related biomarker in their study was the first paper in which voice parameters were used in relation to genetic syndromes. Genetic characteristics of voice in normal people have been elucidated with the location of F0, among others, in ABCC9 genetic variants [4] and confirmed later [6]. The future implementation of voice-related biomarkers heralds a significant paradigm shift, offering enhanced prognostic capabilities for supporting individuals with genetic disabilities, including atypical child development [60].

References

1. Pedersen M, Dinnesen A, Mahmood S. Chapter 4.9 genetic background of voice disorders and genetic perspectives in voice treatment. In: am Zehnhoff-Dinnesen A, Wiskirska-Woźnica B, Neumann K, Nawka T, editors. Phoniatrics I: fundamentals, voice disorders, disorders of language and hearing development. 1st ed. Berlin: Springer; 2020. p. 225–30. (European Manual of Medicine).
2. Nashaat NH, Elrouby I, Zeidan HM, Kilany A, Abdelraouf ER, Hashish AF, Abdelhady HS, ElKeblawy MM, Shadi MS. Childhood apraxia of speech: exploring gluten sensitivity and changes in glutamate and gamma-aminobutyric acid plasma levels. Pediatr Neurol. 2024 Feb;151:104–10. https://doi.org/10.1016/j.pediatrneurol.2023.11.012.

3. Nashaat NH, Meguid NA, Abdelraouf ER, Helmy NA, Dardir AA, Stojanovik V, El-Nofely AA. Linguistic phenotype in a sample of Arabic speaking children with Williams and fragile X syndromes. Biosci Res. 2018;15(2):873–82.
4. Gisladottir RS, Helgason A, Halldorsson BV, Helgason H, Borsky M, Chien YR, et al. Sequence variants affecting voice pitch in humans. Sci Adv. 2023;9(23):eabq2969. https://doi.org/10.1126/sciadv.abq2969.
5. Lechien JR, Geneid A, Bohlender JE, Cantarella G, Avellaneda JC, Desuter G, et al. Consensus for voice quality assessment in clinical practice: guidelines of the European laryngological society and Union of the European Phoniatricians. Eur Arch Otorrinolaringol. 2023 Dec;280(12):5459–73. https://doi.org/10.1007/s00405-023-08211-6.
6. Di Y, Mefford J, Rahmani E, Wang J, Ravi V, Gorla A, et al. Genetic association analysis of human median voice pitch identifies a common locus for tonal and non-tonal languages. Commun Biol. 2024;7(1) https://doi.org/10.1038/s42003-024-06198-2.
7. Luchesi LC, Cavalcanti JC, Lucci TK, David VF, Otta E, Monticelli PF. Zygosity effects on human voice: fundamental frequency analysis of Brazilian twins' speech. Twin Res Hum Genet. 2024 Aug;27(4–5):215–22. https://doi.org/10.1017/thg.2024.33.
8. Mohd Khairuddin KA, Ahmad K, Proehoeman SC, Mohd Ibrahim H, Yan Y. Preliminary findings of vocal fold vibratory characteristics of singers analyzed by laryngeal high-speed Videoendoscopy. J Voice. 2024;S0892-1997(24):00173–5. https://doi.org/10.1016/j.jvoice.2024.06.001.
9. Baum D. Singer's voice quality: genetic or environmental influences? Sci J Lander Coll Arts Sci. 2023;16(2):58–64. Available from: https://touroscholar.touro.edu/sjlcas/vol16/iss2/10
10. Zhang S, Zhao J, Guo Z, Jones JA, Liu P, Liu H. The association between genetic variation in *FOXP2* and sensorimotor control of speech production. Front Neurosci. 2018 Sep;20(12):666. https://doi.org/10.3389/fnins.2018.00666.
11. de Miguel-Luken MJ, Chaves-Conde M, Carnero A. A genetic view of laryngeal cancer heterogeneity. Cell Cycle. 2016;15(9):1202–12. https://doi.org/10.1080/15384101.2016.1156275.
12. Saft C, Jessen J, Hoffmann R, Lukas C, Skodda S. Speech biomarkers in Huntington's disease: a longitudinal follow-up study in Premanifest mutation carriers. J Huntingtons Dis. 2024;13(3):369–73. https://doi.org/10.3233/JHD-240021.
13. Kao TH, Rowe HP, Green JR, Stipancic KL, Sharma N, de Guzman JK, et al. Oral diadochokinetic markers of X-linked dystonia-parkinsonism. Parkinsonism Relat Disord. 2024 Mar;120:105991. https://doi.org/10.1016/j.parkreldis.2024.
14. Calà F, Frassineti L, Sforza E, Onesimo R, D'Alatri L, Manfredi C, et al. Artificial intelligence procedure for the screening of genetic syndromes based on voice characteristics. Bioengineering (Basel). 2023;10(12):1375. https://doi.org/10.3390/bioengineering10121375.
15. O'Brien ARW, Fujiki RB. Prevalence of voice and swallow problems in individuals living with sickle cell disease. Blood. 2023;142(Supplement 1):2514. https://doi.org/10.1182/blood-2023-185284.
16. Semmler M, Kniesburges S, Pelka F, Ensthaler M, Wendler O, Schützenberger A. Influence of reduced saliva production on phonation in patients with ectodermal dysplasia. J Voice. 2023 Nov;37(6):913–23. https://doi.org/10.1016/j.jvoice.2021.06.016.
17. Pelka F, Ensthaler M, Wendler O, Kniesburges S, Schützenberger A, Semmler M. Mechanical parameters based on high-speed Videoendoscopy of the vocal folds in patients with ectodermal dysplasia. J Voice. 2023. S0892–1997(23)00084-X; https://doi.org/10.1016/j.jvoice.2023.02.027.
18. Frassineti L, Calà F, Sforza E, Onesimo R, Leoni C, Lanatà A, et al. Quantitative acoustical analysis of genetic syndromes in the number listing task. Biomed Signal Process Control. 2023;85:104887. https://doi.org/10.1016/j.bspc.2023.104887.
19. Friedman L, Lauber M, Behroozmand R, Fogerty D, Kunecki D, Berry-Kravis E, Klusek J. Atypical vocal quality in women with the FMR1 premutation: an indicator of impaired sensorimotor control. Exp Brain Res. 2023 Aug;241(8):1975–87. https://doi.org/10.1007/s00221-023-06653-2.

20. Jacinto-Scudeiro LA, Rothe-Neves R, Dos Santos VB, Machado GD, Burguêz D, Padovani MMP, et al. Dysarthria in hereditary spastic paraplegia type 4. Clinics (Sao Paulo). 2022;78:100128. https://doi.org/10.1016/j.clinsp.2022.100128.
21. Riad R, Lunven M, Titeux H, Cao XN, Hamet Bagnou J, Lemoine L, et al. Predicting clinical scores in Huntington's disease: a lightweight speech test. J Neurol. 2022 Sep;269(9):5008–21. https://doi.org/10.1007/s00415-022-11148-1.
22. Cordella C, Gutz SE, Eshghi M, Stipancic KL, Schliep M, Dickerson BC, Green JR. Acoustic and kinematic assessment of motor speech impairment in patients with suspected four-repeat Tauopathies. J Speech Lang Hear Res. 2022;65(11):4112–32. https://doi.org/10.1044/2022_JSLHR-22-00177.
23. Pokorny FB, Schmitt M, Egger M, Bartl-Pokorny KD, Zhang D, Schuller BW, et al. Automatic vocalisation-based detection of fragile X syndrome and Rett syndrome. Sci Rep. 2022;12(1) https://doi.org/10.1038/s41598-022-17203-1.
24. Hseu AF, Spencer GP, Jo S, Clark R, Nuss RC. Laryngeal pathologies in dysphonic children with down syndrome. Int J Pediatr Otorhinolaryngol. 2022 Jun;157:111118. https://doi.org/10.1016/j.ijporl.2022.111118.
25. Singh R. Connecting human voice profiling to genomics: a predictive algorithm for linking speech phenotypes to genetic microdeletion syndromes. bioRxiv. Cold Spring Harbor Laboratory; 2022. https://doi.org/10.1101/2022.05.23.493126.
26. de Andrade BMR, Valença EHO, Salvatori R, Neto OLA, Souza AHO, Oliveira AHA, et al. Art and science: impact of semioccluded vocal tract exercises and choral singing on quality of life in subjects with congenital GH deficiency. Arch Endocrinol Metab. 2022;66(2):198–205. https://doi.org/10.20945/2359-3997000000449.
27. Sacconi S. Facial and vocal recognition as a decision support tool for neuromuscular diseases: the FACENMD project. J Neuromuscul Dis. 2022; https://doi.org/10.3233/JND-229001.
28. Lowell SY, Kelley RT, Dischinat N, Monahan M, Hosbach-Cannon CJ, Colton RH, et al. Clinical features of essential voice tremor and associations with tremor severity and response to Octanoic acid treatment. Laryngoscope. 2021;131(11) https://doi.org/10.1002/lary.29558.
29. Kosztyła-Hojna B, Borys J, Zdrojkowski M, Duchnowska E, Kraszewska A, Wasilewska D, Zweier C, Midro AT. Phoniatric, audiological, Orodental and speech problems in a boy with cardio-Facio-cutaneous syndrome type 3 (CFC 3) due to a pathogenic variant in *MAP2K1* – case study. Appl Clin Genet. 2021 Sep;6(14):389–98. https://doi.org/10.2147/TACG.S316215.
30. Neves PCR, Toralles MBP, Scarpel RD. Perfil Vocal de Indivíduos 46, XX com Hiperplasia Adrenal Congênita. Codas. 2021;33(5) https://doi.org/10.1590/2317-1782/20202018260.
31. Hidalgo-De la Guía I, Garayzábal-Heinze E, Gómez-Vilda P, Martínez-Olalla R, Palacios-Alonso D. Acoustic analysis of phonation in children with smith-Magenis syndrome. Front Hum Neurosci. 2021;15:661392. https://doi.org/10.3389/fnhum.2021.661392.
32. La Guía IHD, Garayzábal E, Gómez-Vilda P, Palacios-Alonso D. Specificities of phonation biomechanics in down syndrome children. Biomed Signal Process Control. 2020 Oct;8(63):102219. https://doi.org/10.1016/j.bspc.2020.102219.
33. Song SA, Go CL, Acuna PB, De Guzman JKP, Sharma N, Song PC. Progressive decline in voice and voice-related quality of life in X-linked dystonia parkinsonism. J Voice. 2023 Jan;37(1):134–8. https://doi.org/10.1016/j.jvoice.2020.11.014.
34. Krishnamurthy R, Ramani SA. Aerodynamic and acoustic characteristics of voice in children with down syndrome-a systematic review. Int J Pediatr Otorhinolaryngol. 2020 Jun;133:109946. https://doi.org/10.1016/j.ijporl.2020.109946.
35. Moya-Mendez ME, Madden LL, Ruckart KW, Downes KM, Cook JF, Snively BM, et al. Auditory-perceptual voice and speech evaluation in ATP1A3 positive patients. J Clin Neurosci. 2020 Nov;81:133–8. https://doi.org/10.1016/j.jocn.2020.09.007.
36. Carraro L, Carecchio M, Antonini A. Phenotypic characterization of a cohort of patients affected by laryngeal dystonia: a monocentric study. 2020.
37. Sobuś A, Baumert B, Pawlukowska W, Gołąb-Janowska M, Paczkowska E, Wełnicka A, et al. Humoral influence of repeated lineage-negative stem/progenitor cell administration

on articulatory functions in ALS patients. Stem Cells Int. 2020;2020:8888271. https://doi.org/10.1155/2020/8888271.
38. Pebbili GK, Kashyap R, J R, Karike A, Navya A. Laryngeal aerodynamic analysis of glottal Valving in children with down syndrome. J Voice. 2021 Jan;35(1):156.e15–21. https://doi.org/10.1016/j.jvoice.2019.05.011.
39. Bartier S, Bodez D, Kharoubi M, Canouï-Poitrine F, Chatelin V, Henrion C, et al. Pharyngolaryngeal involvement in systemic amyloidosis with cardiac involvement: a prospective observational study. Amyloid. 2019 Dec;26(4):216–24. https://doi.org/10.1080/13506129.2019.1646639.
40. Ali L, Zhu C, Zhang Z, Liu Y. Automated detection of Parkinson's disease based on multiple types of sustained phonations using linear discriminant analysis and genetically optimized neural network. IEEE J Transl Eng Health Med. 2019;7:2000410. https://doi.org/10.1109/JTEHM.2019.2940900.
41. Kleim K, Simonyan K, Ball T. Objective evaluation criteria for diagnosis of spasmodic dysphonia [abstract]. Mov Disord. 2019;34(suppl 2) Available from: https://www.mdsabstracts.org/abstract/objective-evaluation-criteria-for-diagnosis-of-spasmodic-dysphonia/
42. Spencer KA, Dawson M. Dysarthria profiles in adults with hereditary ataxia. Am J Speech Lang Pathol. 2019;28(2S):915–24. https://doi.org/10.1044/2018_AJSLP-MSC18-18-0114.
43. Khodadoust M, Pourzaki M, Ghelichi L. Speech difficulties in Joubert syndrome. Koomesh. 2019;21(2):387–90.
44. Sebastián-Lázaro D, Brun-Gasca C, Fornieles-Deu A. Voz y Habla de los Niños con Síndrome de Deleción de 22q11. Rev Neurol. 2019;68(3):99–106. https://doi.org/10.33588/rn.6803.2018279.
45. Nevler N, Ash S, Irwin DJ, Liberman M, Grossman M. Validated automatic speech biomarkers in primary progressive aphasia. Ann Clin Transl Neurol. 2018;6(1):4–14. https://doi.org/10.1002/acn3.653.
46. Ebert B, Sidman J, Morrell N, Roby BB. Congenital and iatrogenic laryngeal and vocal abnormalities in patients with 22q11.2 deletion. Int J Pediatr Otorhinolaryngol. 2018 Jun;109:17–20. https://doi.org/10.1016/j.ijporl.2018.03.006.
47. Jackowska J, Klimza H, Zagozda N, Remacle M, Wojnowski W, Piersiala K, Wierzbicka M. Thyroplasty in unilateral vocal fold paresis with coexisting hereditary hemorrhagic telenagiectasia: a case report. Medicine (Baltimore). 2018 Oct;97(41):e12727. https://doi.org/10.1097/MD.0000000000012727.
48. Vogel AP, Rommel N, Oettinger A, Stoll LH, Kraus EM, Gagnon C, et al. Coordination and timing deficits in speech and swallowing in autosomal recessive spastic ataxia of Charlevoix-Saguenay (ARSACS). J Neurol. 2018 Sep;265(9):2060–70. https://doi.org/10.1007/s00415-018-8950-4.
49. Konstantopoulos K, Zamba-Papanicolaou E, Christodoulou K. Quantification of dysarthrophonia in a Cypriot family with autosomal recessive hereditary spastic paraplegia associated with a homozygous SPG11 mutation. Neurol Sci. 2018 Sep;39(9):1547–50. https://doi.org/10.1007/s10072-018-3453-8.
50. Szklanny K, Gubrynowicz R, Tylki-Szymańska A. Voice alterations in patients with Morquio A syndrome. J Appl Genet. 2018 Feb;59(1):73–80. https://doi.org/10.1007/s13353-017-0421-6.
51. Demopoulos C, Kothare H, Mizuiri D, Henderson-Sabes J, Fregeau B, Tjernagel J, et al. Abnormal speech motor control in individuals with 16p11.2 deletions. Sci Rep. 2018;8(1):1274. https://doi.org/10.1038/s41598-018-19751-x.
52. Hidalgo I, Gómez Vilda P, Garayzábal E. Biomechanical description of phonation in children affected by Williams syndrome. J Voice. 2018 Jul;32(4):515.e15–28. https://doi.org/10.1016/j.jvoice.2017.07.002.
53. Vogel AP, Rommel N, Oettinger A, Horger M, Krumm P, Kraus EM, et al. Speech and swallowing abnormalities in adults with POLG associated ataxia (POLG-A). Mitochondrion. 2017 Nov;37:1–7. https://doi.org/10.1016/j.mito.2017.06.002.

54. Vogel AP, Wardrop MI, Folker JE, Synofzik M, Corben LA, Delatycki MB, Awan SN. Voice in Friedreich Ataxia. J Voice. 2017 Mar;31(2):243.e9–243.e19. https://doi.org/10.1016/j.jvoice.2016.04.015.
55. Poujois A, Pernon M, Trocello JM, Woimant F. Dystonic dysarthria in Wilson disease: efficacy of zolpidem. Front Neurol. 2017;8:559. https://doi.org/10.3389/fneur.2017.00559.
56. Hintze JM, Ludlow CL, Bansberg SF, Adler CH, Lott DG. Spasmodic dysphonia: a review. Part 1: pathogenic factors. Otolaryngol Head Neck Surg. 2017 Oct;157(4):551–7. https://doi.org/10.1177/0194599817728521.
57. Turner SJ, Brown A, Arpone M, Anderson V, Morgan AT, Scheffer IE. Dysarthria and broader motor speech deficits in Dravet syndrome. Neurology. 2017;88(8):743–9. https://doi.org/10.1212/WNL.0000000000003635.
58. Wolf AE, Mourão L, França MC Jr, Machado Júnior AJ, Crespo AN. Phonoarticulation in spinocerebellar ataxia type 3. Eur Arch Otorrinolaringol. 2017 Feb;274(2):1139–45. https://doi.org/10.1007/s00405-016-4240-x.
59. Montazeri M, Khoddami M, Zamani Rad M, Mazaheri S, Alizadeh M, Jalaei S. Voice acoustic and perceptual features in lipoid proteinosis: a report of two cases. J Mazandaran Univ Med Sci. 2017;26(145):414–20. Available from: http://jmums.mazums.ac.ir/article-1-9502-en.html
60. Pedersen M. Normal development of voice. 2nd ed. Springer Verlag; 2024. https://doi.org/10.1007/978-3-031-42391-8.
61. Pedersen M. Artificial intelligence for screening voice disorders: aspects of risk factors: research article. Am J Med Clin Res Rev. 2025 Feb;4(2):1–8. https://doi.org/10.58372/2835-6276.1254.

Open Access This chapter is licensed under the terms of the Creative Commons Attribution-NonCommercial-NoDerivatives 4.0 International License (http://creativecommons.org/licenses/by-nc-nd/4.0/), which permits any noncommercial use, sharing, distribution and reproduction in any medium or format, as long as you give appropriate credit to the original author(s) and the source, provide a link to the Creative Commons license and indicate if you modified the licensed material. You do not have permission under this license to share adapted material derived from this chapter or parts of it.

The images or other third party material in this chapter are included in the chapter's Creative Commons license, unless indicated otherwise in a credit line to the material. If material is not included in the chapter's Creative Commons license and your intended use is not permitted by statutory regulation or exceeds the permitted use, you will need to obtain permission directly from the copyright holder.

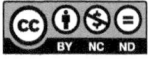

Optical Coherence Tomography and Voice-Related Biomarkers

13

Mette Pedersen ⓘ

13.1 Introduction

Forward steps have been made for the possibilities of Optical Coherence Tomography (OCT) since 1991, when the method was presented in ophthalmology [1]. It is possible to make many diagnoses even on a cellular level with OCT corresponding to the development of the area of molecular biology [2–5]. Another aspect is the use of artificial intelligence to automate diagnoses and identify disorders with OCT [6–12]. Research on voice-related biomarkers should follow the development of OCT in other areas where analyses are possible in commercial equipment [13, 14]. Apart from classification and eventual documentation of the effect of treatment, the function of the tissue is of special interest, refined with Ultra-High-Resolution OCT (UHR-OCT) in many parts of animals and the human body [15–18]. Park et al. [19] compared OCT with UHR-OCT in esophageal neoplasia and found, on average, a two times greater contrast and more detailed visualization of tissue microstructure, a sharper definition of surface signal intensity, and clearer delineation of mucosal glands and layer effacement. Wolfgang et al. [20] used UHR-OCT to optimize the investigation of automated thin multilayered pharmaceutical coating resolutions. Pedersen [21] commented on the possibilities for UHR-OCT in the larynx combined with high-speed films.

In laryngology, classification of benign and malignant disorders includes the vocal folds but also the arytenoid regions, where a difference between reflux, allergy, and infection is possible based on deviations of the tissue [22–24]. The quantitative diagnosis of edema of the vocal folds could be a big step forward. It is possible to measure the thickness of the epithelium and lamina propria of the vocal folds with and without intonation, and the movements of the cover layers can be presented. The impact of these measurements has interesting perspectives for

M. Pedersen (✉)
The Medical Center, Copenhagen, Denmark
e-mail: M.f.pedersen@dadlnet.dk

© The Author(s) 2026
M. Pedersen et al. (eds.), *Voice-related Biomarkers*,
https://doi.org/10.1007/978-3-032-03134-1_13

voice-related biomarkers. In surgery, OCT gives a clearer view of how much tissue to remove [25–29]. Documentation of rehabilitation after treatment can be done with the classification and function of the tissue, coordinated with the other voice-related biomarkers. The development and function of the vocal folds during normal speech and singing have been analyzed in recent years with OCT by Garcia et al. [30, 31] and Benboujja et al. [32, 33]. OCT and UHR-OCT are possibilities for describing the movements of the vocal folds as well as measuring the thickness of the epithelium and lamina propria during function. The tutorial overview aimed to show research results that are ready for commercial types of equipment [34] even in laryngology. Many supplementary software programs can be taken over from other specialties for analysis in the larynx.

13.2 Material

OCT possibilities in laryngology have been presented in the introduction. OCT corresponds to an ultrasound examination based on laser light instead of ultrasound. OCT can be a supplement and further developmental option of ultrasound analyses. The OCT technology was developed as a Time-Domain OCT system (TD-OCT) in ophthalmology, dependent on a moving mirror as a reference arm, using a photodiode for analysis of laser light. The weak point of this technique is the need to move the reference mirror to obtain images from various depths. It creates a speed limit and can lead to motion artifacts in the scanned image. This is crucial in laryngology, where the vocal folds oscillate with a mean frequency of 110 Hz for men and 220 Hz for women in average speech. Fourier Domain systems (FD-OCT), such as Spectral Domain OCT (SD-OCT) and Swept Source OCT (SS-OCT), give solutions with a fixed mirror as a reference arm; SD-OCT emits the entire needed laser range of wavelength all the time. Whereas SS-OCT uses a tunable laser to emit the same wavelength in sequence and synchronizes with the diode [35, 36]. Highly developed laser light sources include superluminescent diodes that give a high axial resolution in the tissues.

Various methods for OCT setups exist. In Fig. 13.1, one of the most advanced UHR-OCTs is introduced with a high penetration depth. When it comes to scanning probes, one of the published ones is presented in Fig. 13.2, with a working distance of 7–10 cm. The image speed is 200 frames per second (fps). An interesting pharynx tissue presentation in Fig. 13.3 is based on an axial depth of 1300 nm; the axial resolution is 20 µm and the lateral resolution is 25 µm, with TD-OCT 10 fps forward-looking contact probe. The images presented in Fig. 13.3 are based on a time-domain setup with a movable mirror as a reference arm. Later studies use SS-OCT with a fixed mirror as a reference arm and a broadband swept source. Similar pictures can be taken of the larynx mucosa in the clinic with a relevant future commercial probe. The aspects include the whole larynx, the vocal folds, and also specifically the arytenoid regions. In Fig. 13.3, *a classification* of disorders is presented. But in Fig. 13.4, the possibilities of *function* analyses with Python software are an aspect where the hardware and software are *ready for commercialization*. Laser ablation of

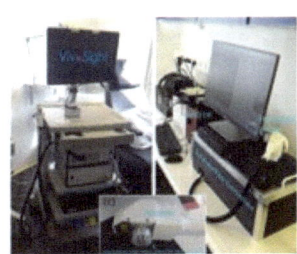
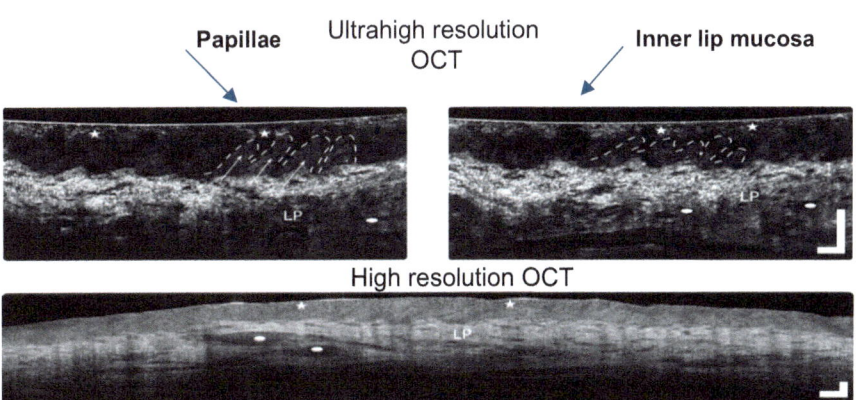

Fig. 13.1 Testing the dermatological UHR-OCT system for the oral cavity. This figure shows that with UHR-OCT, the papillae and details of the mucosa are well presented. This is also the case for capillaries, glands, and various cell types [23, 36]. (Reproduced from Israelsen et al. [36]. With permission from Ugeskrift for Lægers videnskabelige redaktionssekretariat)

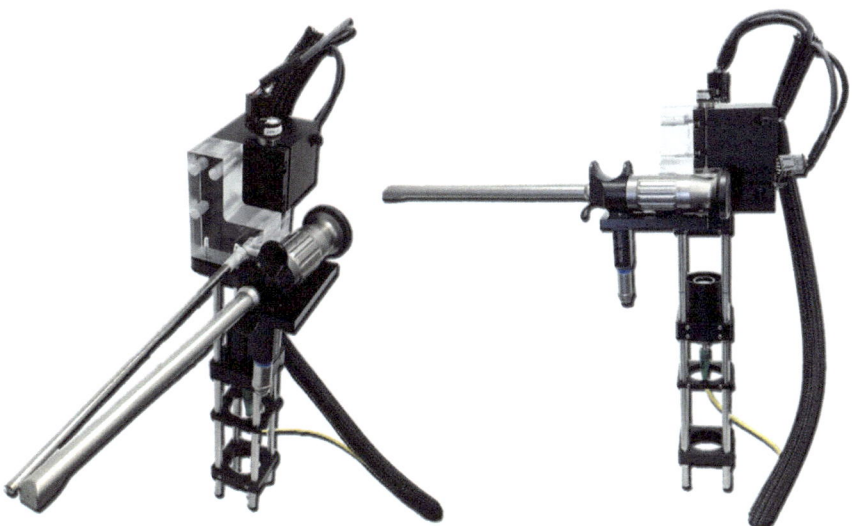

Fig. 13.2 Endoscope OCT systems have been developed. SS-OCT, 1310 nm, 200 kHz VCSEL, Working distance: 7–10 cm, Axial resolution: 9.3 μm, Lateral resolution: 100 μm, Pixel resolution: 5.9 μm, Imaging speed: 200 fps [37]. (Copyright: Coughlan et al. [37], redistributed under the terms of the Creative Commons Attribution License (CC BY 4.0))

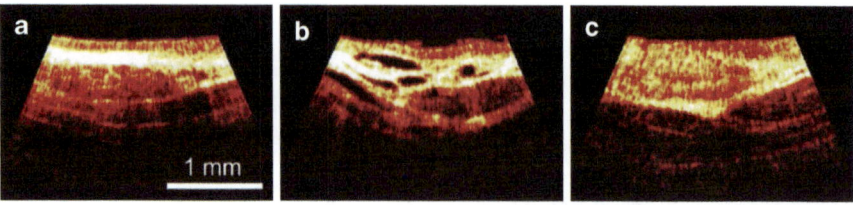

Fig. 13.3 OCT images of the pharynx mucosa. (**a**) *Normal*: The upper layer is characterized by a moderate signal level corresponding to stratified squamous epithelium, while the lower layer with a high signal level corresponds to lamina propria with a high content of elastin fibers. In the submucous layer glands and lymphoid elements are manifested in OCT images by irregularly shaped areas. (**b**) *Chronic pharyngitis*: Catarrhal form of pharyngitis, persistent diffuse congestion of the veins accompanied by pronounced edema of tissues is observed leading to the disintegration of morphological structures and an increase in the volume of lymphoid tissue with building of subepithelial cysts. (**c**) *After therapy*: Therapy is accompanied by water crystallization manifested in OCT images by the disappearance of low-signal areas and a balance of the signal level in the upper layers. Use of TD-OCT forward-looking contact mini-probe with an axial depth of 1300 nm, axial resolution in air of 20 μm, and lateral resolution of 25 μm. (Used with permission of Walter de Gruyter and Company, from Meller et al. [38]; permission conveyed through Copyright Clearance Center, Inc.)

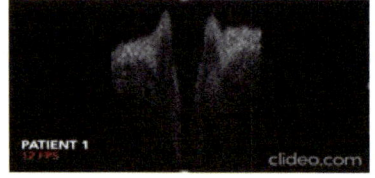

During resting state, in males the epithelium state was 106 ± 49 μm, and the lamina propria 367 ± 197 μm in females, it was 66 ± 24 μm and 595 ± 179 μm respectively. *During phonation* in males, the epithelium state was 81 ± 35 μm, and the lamina propria 376 ± 130 μm in females, it was 79 ± 38 μm and 522 ± 220 μm respectively	**Propagation with different amplitudes.** **For the X-axis horizontal wave**: 30 points were distributed equidistantly along the width of the superior contour of each vocal fold. **For the Y-axis vertical wave**: with consecutive phonation over a period of at least 3 s, the vertical mucosal wave can be visualized and measured. **The Green lines** visually demarcate the displacement vector between the 30 equidistant points along the superior surface of each segmentation **The Yellow** and **orange lines** show two epithelium segmentations from consecutive image frames.

Fig. 13.4 Vocal fold mucosa propagation. The vertical displacement was 1.38 mm in males and 1.24 mm in females. This figure shows the calculated epithelium and lamina propria during rest and phonation. The calculation of the propagation of the amplitude is illustrated. (Copyright: Sharma et al. [39], redistributed under the terms of the Creative Commons Attribution License (CC BY 4.0))

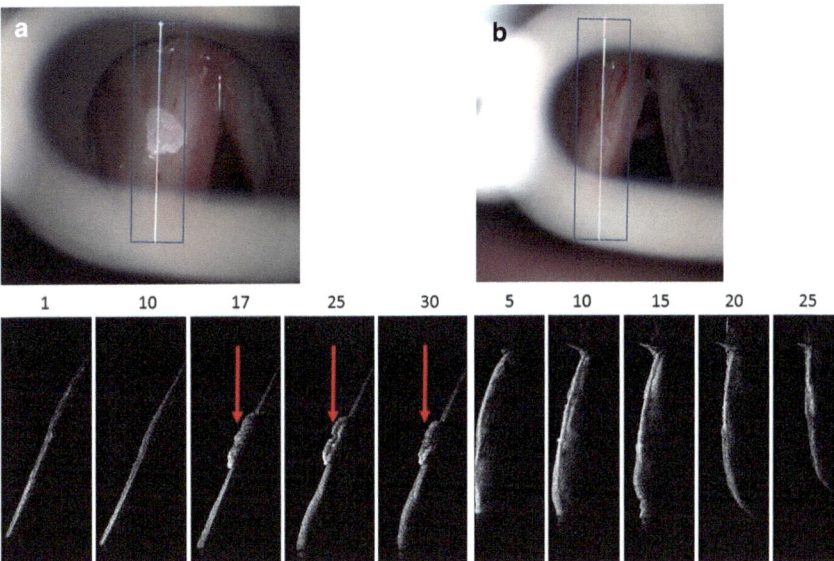

Fig. 13.5 OCT of a hyperkeratotic lesion in an outpatient setting. OCT images of a hyperkeratotic lesion in the left vocal fold. On the left, panel (**a**) it shows the vocal fold before laser ablation with the corresponding OCT image slides taken from lateral (1) to medial (30), clearly depicting the thickening of the epithelium (17, 25, 30), as indicated by the red arrow. On the right, panel (**b**) it shows the vocal fold after laser ablation with the corresponding OCT image slides, again taken from the lateral (5) to medial (25) side, depicting a smooth epithelial surface. OCT, optical coherence tomography. (Copyright: Witting et al. [40], redistributed under the terms of the Creative Commons Attribution License (CC BY 4.0))

tissue on the vocal folds can be performed with the help of OCT, as presented in Fig. 13.5. The figures are discussed in detail below.

13.3 Methods

OCT has been used for vocal folds in direct contact. The problem with practical routine clinical indirect use is the distance between probes in the pharynx. Studies hereof are conducted at several research centers. Its use in other areas of the larynx is also of interest. The newest aspect of clinical tissue diagnostics is UHR-OCT. If probe-tissue contact is possible, ultra-high, fine axial, and lateral resolutions can be obtained. In Fig. 13.1, the apparatus developed by Israelsen et al. [16] is used for the contact UHR-OCT. The cell details are presented, as well as the glands and capillaries. It was compared with a commercial program in dermatology, showing the contact layers of the mucosa. Table 13.1 shows the differences between UHR-OCT and commercial OCT (C-OCT) measurements. The actual optical resolution in the tissue is smaller in μm, but the operating wavelength is larger.

Table 13.1 Comparison between UHR-OCT and commercial OCT (C-OCT)

System feature	C-OCT	UHR-OCT
Operating wavelength (nm)	1305	1270 (1070–1470)
Axial optical resolution in tissue (µm)	<5	2.2
Lateral optical resolution in air (µm)	<7.5	6
Depth of focus (mm)	1	0.05 (Rayleigh length)
Axial digital sampling in tissue (µm)	4.12	1.46
Lateral digital sampling (µm)	4.41	2.93
Scanning area (mm × mm)	4 × 4	3 × 3
Optical average power applied (mW)	5	5

Copyright: Israelsen et al. [16] Optical Society of America under the terms of the OSA Open Access Publishing Agreement
The operating wavelengths as well as the optical resolutions

It is possible to show the vertical and horizontal details in live mode and even present a 3D stack with isotropic cellular resolution in direct skin contact. The commercial setup used for skin disorders is Damae Medical [14].

Another commercial skin analysis presents the capillary flow as supplementary information [13]. Long-range in vivo SS-OCT has been presented as a useful tool in the mouth for diagnosis of infection as well as documentation of treatment effect [41]: Anatomic and microvascular imaging of human oral mucosa tissue is presented. "*Qualitative assessment of the structure characteristics (i.e., collagen fibrosis, volume of salivary glands, and tissue scattering) during wound healing delineates the anatomical lesion development accompanied by tissue inflammation. Quantitative assessment of the vasculature network (i.e., capillary loop density and vessel morphological orientations) revealed pathological and nutritional underpinnings of microcirculation for oral lesion recovery. Specifically, the progression of oral capillary angiogenesis, indicated by elevations in capillary loop density, occurs within 12 hours of disease onset and peaks at day 7 thereafter, which provides invaluable information for the time course of therapeutic treatment*" [41]. This shows the potential movement of oral cavity OCT toward clinical use at a high level. UHR-OCT will also optimize the findings in the larynx [23, 36].

In Fig. 13.2, an OCT system for vocal fold analysis is presented [42]. The setup can work with a probe in real-time in the pharynx at 7–10 cm from the vocal folds. This illustrates that the setup can be used with the aspect of biomarking in the clinic, not only for vocal folds but also for other parts, including the arytenoid regions.

13.4 Results

As shown in Fig. 13.3, a forward-looking TD-OCT mini-probe was used with an axial depth of 1300 nm, an axial resolution in air of 20 µm, a lateral resolution of 25 µm, and 10 fps [38]. A picture of the pharynx is used here to show the possibilities in the larynx. In this case, chronic pharyngitis with hypertrophic mucosa and diffuse congestion of veins was accompanied by pronounced edema of the tissue, with clear changes after therapy by the disappearance of low-signal areas and a balance of the signal levels of the upper layers.

OCT can be used with machine learning for cancer detection in the larynx with preprocessing of the OCT pictures with normalization, cropping, and data augmentation. After that, deep learning layers in a convolutional network can classify the tissue into different groups, supporting the physician's discussion: malignant, benign, and unclear results of classification [40]. Gessert et al. [43] present a clear picture of differences in OCT between normal tissue and cancer tissue using the deep learning models ResNet18, DenseNet121, and SE-ResNeXt50.

Figure 13.4 shows a picture of a film based on the rigid probe from Fig. 13.2. The margins of the vocal folds are seen, and the epithelium as well as the lamina propria can be differentiated. The films were preprocessed as shown in the flowchart; the major steps are indicated, and Python was used for the analysis [39, supplement]. With relevant software, the analysis can be combined with other voice-related biomarkers. The function of the vocal folds is analyzed with the vertical displacement during intonation being 1.38 mm in males and 1.24 mm in females, based on 30 points distributed equidistantly along the superior contour of each vocal fold. The epithelial state of the epithelium and lamina propria is also of interest, being 106 and 367 µm vs. 81 and 376 µm in males and 66 and 595 vs. 79 and 522 µm in females during the resting state and phonation, respectively. Standard deviations are given in Fig. 13.4.

The flowchart of the initial image-processing steps

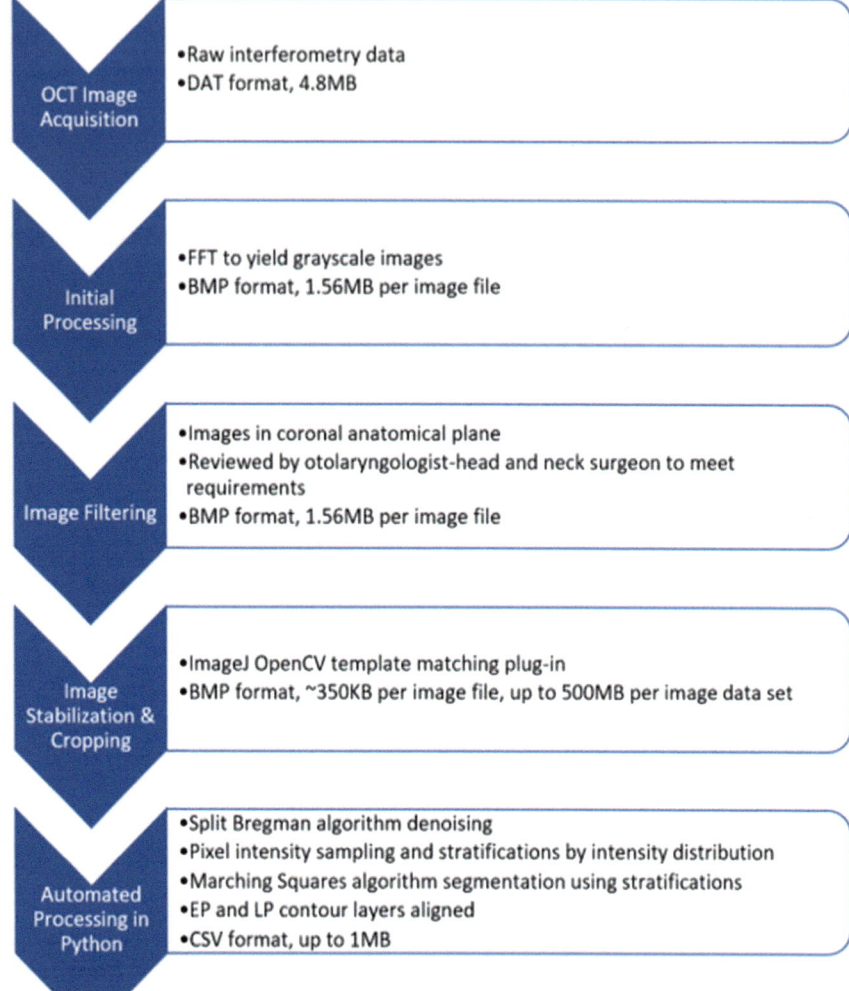

The flowchart shows the preprocessing. Python software was used for the analysis, as shown in Fig. 13.4. (Copyright: Sharma et al. [39], redistributed under the terms of the Creative Commons Attribution License (CC BY 4.0))

In Fig. 13.5, a clinical situation in an outpatient setting is shown with a new OCT microscope (OP MedT OCT camera) [40] showing how a hyperkeratotic lesion on the left vocal fold can be removed and the epithelial border cleared up on OCT. In principle, the OCT is functioning here as a voice-related biomarker. The latest approach is a probe for high-speed URH-OCT to provide clinical evidence for targeting diseases: edema and detailed benign and malignant lesions [23, 36].

13.5 Discussion

In Fig. 13.1, the setup for UHR-OCT is shown to be usable in direct contact with the mucosa. The mucosa of the lower lip is used, as it resembles the larynx mucosa. A commercial probe for the larynx is under construction The UHR-OCT potential lies in the better definition of tissues, capillaries, glands, papillae, and various kinds of cells. A planned probe is rigid, considering the distance of around 10 cm from the uvula to the vocal folds in awake patients. These results would give a better clinical basis for OCT as a supplementary voice-related biomarker.

The scientific literature includes many papers on the analysis of finer parts of tissues using machine learning. Therefore, machine learning is ideal, as presented in Fig. 13.4. Also, other OCT systems in ENT are of interest, e.g., for the nose [44]. Experience, especially by dermatologists and ophthalmologists with deep learning, can be transferred to the area of voice-related biomarkers and other parts of the field of oto-rhino-laryngology.

For UHR-OCT, the SS-OCT-200 kHz rigid side-viewing endoscope based on VCSEL is of great interest with its working distance of 7–10 cm and axial resolution of 9.3 µm, with high imaging speeds as described at the bottom of the figure. We thereby can establish not only a classification of disorders but also show function and deviation in tissue pathology. OCT systems are of interest to show allergies and infections, as well as reflux tissue reactions, as shown in Fig. 13.3 for the pharynx. We have today no commercial tools in vivo objectively and decisively to measure tissue pathology in the larynx; therefore, OCT is of interest for randomized controlled trials of treatments for malignant as well as benign neoplasms.

The aspects of the advanced voice-related biomarker technology are shown in Fig. 13.4 [39]. UHR-OCT can show many more details. This is the case for the epithelium and lamina propria, and measuring Reincke's space per se in the vocal folds may be possible. Exact films of the regions of interest (ROI) can be considered [45]. The demands for these analyses have not been made clear enough to the public, probably because the research results have not been described broadly and generally enough. The value of OCT for operations on the vocal folds cannot be presented better than that in Fig. 13.5, where the epithelium after removal of hyperkeratosis is intact on OCT.

It must be made clear to the public that we are working without evidence when it comes to IN VIVO tissue pathology in the larynx, apart from some cancer forms. Pharmacological medicine needs classification and functional evidence from randomized controlled studies to show the medical effects on allergies, infection, and reflux in the upper airways [20, 21]. Few papers are written on this topic [46]. UHR-OCT is optimal for resolving these issues. As shown in Fig. 13.5, regular margins and epithelium can be defined with or without a machine learning approach and documentation of treatment, and voice-related biomarkers can be supplemented as in other fields, like ophthalmology and dermatology.

13.6 Conclusion

An overview of the clinical perspectives of OCT and UHR-OCT related to the previously referenced voice-related biomarkers has been made. With help from commercial firms, tissue diagnostics can become possible for the classification of many benign disorders, as well as for refining diagnoses of malignancy, using the right probes. The best probe for indirect laryngoscopy to date is an SS-OCT, 200 kHz, vertical-cavity-surface-emitting-laser with 200 fps and an axial resolution of 9.3 μm. The UHR-OCT potential lies in the better definition of the tissues, capillaries, glands, papillae, and various kinds of cells. Aspects are vast—for example, in prognoses after treatment of malignancy, not only for reflux, allergies, and infections, but also for professional singers and speakers.

Acknowledgments Thank you to Christian Frederik Larsen for inspiring discussions during the preparation of the manuscript and Vitus Girelli Meiner for great help.

References

1. Huang D, Swanson EA, Lin CP, Schuman JS, Stinson WG, Chang W, Hee MR, Flotte T, Gregory K, Puliafito CA, et al. Optical coherence tomography. Science. 1991;254(5035):1178–81. https://doi.org/10.1126/science.1957169.
2. Aumann S, Donner S, Fischer J, Müller F. Chapter 3: Optical coherence tomography (OCT): principle and technical realization. In: Bille JF, editor. High-resolution imaging in microscopy and ophthalmology: new frontiers in biomedical optics. Cham: Springer; 2019. https://doi.org/10.1007/978-3-030-16638-0_3.
3. Thiboutot J, Yuan W, Park HC, Li D, Loube J, Mitzner W, et al. Visualization and validation of the microstructures in the airway wall in vivo using diffractive optical coherence tomography. Acad Radiol. 2022;29(11):1623–30. https://doi.org/10.1016/j.acra.2022.01.008.
4. Leichtle A, Penxova Z, Kempin T, Leffers D, Ahrens M, König P, et al. Dynamic microscopic optical coherence tomography as a new diagnostic tool for otitis media. Photonics. 2023;10(6):685. https://doi.org/10.3390/photonics10060685.
5. Schie IW, Placzek F, Knorr F, Cordero E, Wurster LM, Hermann GG, et al. Morpho-molecular signal correlation between optical coherence tomography and Raman spectroscopy for superior image interpretation and clinical diagnosis. Sci Rep. 2021;11(1):9951. https://doi.org/10.1038/s41598-021-89188-2.
6. Pedersen M, Mahmood S. Future aspects of cellular and molecular research in clinical voice treatment aspects of optical coherence tomography. Proc SPIE. 2015;9303:93031R. https://doi.org/10.1117/12.2076378.
7. Ronneberger O, Fischer P, Brox T. U-Net: convolutional networks for biomedical image segmentation. In: Navab N, Hornegger J, Wells WM, Frangi AF, editors. Medical image computing and computer-assisted intervention – MICCAI 2015, Lecture notes in computer science, vol. 9351. Cham: Springer; 2015. p. 234–41. https://doi.org/10.1007/978-3-319-24574-4_28.
8. Ran AR, Tham CC, Chan PP, Cheng CY, Tham YC, Rim TH, Cheung CY. Deep learning in glaucoma with optical coherence tomography: a review. Eye (Lond). 2021;35(1):188–201. https://doi.org/10.1038/s41433-020-01191-5.
9. Muchuchuti S, Viriri S. Retinal disease detection using deep learning techniques: a comprehensive review. J Imaging. 2023;9(4):84. https://doi.org/10.3390/jimaging9040084.

10. Movahhedi M, Liu XY, Geng B, Elemans C, Xue Q, Wang JX, Zheng X. Predicting 3D soft tissue dynamics from 2D imaging using physics informed neural networks. Commun Biol. 2023;6(1):541. https://doi.org/10.1038/s42003-023-04914-y.
11. Munro P. Guest edited collection: quantitative and computational techniques in optical coherence tomography. Sci Rep. 2022;12(1):11808. https://doi.org/10.1038/s41598-022-15424-y.
12. Del Amor R, Morales S, Colomer A, Mogensen M, Jensen M, Israelsen NM, Bang O, Naranjo V. Automatic segmentation of epidermis and hair follicles in optical coherence tomography images of normal skin by convolutional neural networks. Front Med (Lausanne). 2020;7:220. https://doi.org/10.3389/fmed.2020.00220.
13. Deegan AJ, Wang RK. Microvascular imaging of the skin. Phys Med Biol. 2019;64(7):07TR01. https://doi.org/10.1088/1361-6560/ab03f1.
14. Damae Medical, 14 Rue Sthrau, 75013 Paris, France. https://damae-medical.com/.
15. Götzinger E, Baumann B, Pircher M, Hitzenberger CK. Polarization maintaining fiber based ultra-high resolution spectral domain polarization sensitive optical coherence tomography. Opt Express. 2009;17(25):22704–17. https://doi.org/10.1364/OE.17.022704.
16. Israelsen NM, Maria M, Mogensen M, Bojesen S, Jensen M, Haedersdal M, Podoleanu A, Bang O. The value of ultrahigh resolution OCT in dermatology – delineating the dermoepidermal junction, capillaries in the dermal papillae and vellus hairs. Biomed Opt Express. 2018;9(5):2240–65. https://doi.org/10.1364/BOE.9.002240.
17. Israelsen NM, Petersen CR, Barh A, Jain D, Jensen M, Hannesschläger G, Tidemand-Lichtenberg P, Pedersen C, Podoleanu A, Bang O. Real-time high-resolution mid-infrared optical coherence tomography. Light Sci Appl. 2019;8:11. https://doi.org/10.1038/s41377-019-0122-5.
18. Al-Qazwini Z, Ko ZYG, Mehta K, Chen N. Ultrahigh-speed line-scan SD-OCT for four-dimensional in vivo imaging of small animal models. Biomed Opt Express. 2018;9(3):1216–28. https://doi.org/10.1364/BOE.9.001216.
19. Park HC, Kamboj AK, Leggett CL, Li D, Wang KK, Li X. Comparative study of conventional and ultrahigh-resolution optical coherence tomography imaging in esophageal neoplasia. Tech Innov Gastrointest Endosc. 2022;24(3):312–3. https://doi.org/10.1016/j.tige.2022.01.005.
20. Wolfgang M, Kern A, Deng S, Stranzinger S, Liu M, Drexler W, et al. Ultra-high-resolution optical coherence tomography for the investigation of thin multilayered pharmaceutical coatings. Int J Pharm. 2023;643:123096. https://doi.org/10.1016/j.ijpharm.2023.123096.
21. Pedersen M. Ultra-high-resolution (UHR) optical coherence tomography (OCT) in the upper airways: aspect of combined high-speed films and UHR OCT in the larynx. Int J Clin Exp Otolaryngol. 2019;5:101–5. https://doi.org/10.19070/2572-732x-1900018.
22. Paderno A, Gennarini F, Sordi A, Montenegro C, Lancini D, Villani FP, et al. Artificial intelligence in clinical endoscopy: insights in the field of videomics. Front Surg. 2022;9:933297. https://doi.org/10.3389/fsurg.2022.933297.
23. Israelsen NM, Jensen M, Jønsson AO, Pedersen M. Ultrahigh resolution optical coherence tomography for detecting tissue abnormalities of the oral and laryngeal mucosa: a preliminary study. In: Proceedings of 11th international workshop on models and analysis of vocal emissions for biomedical applications. Florence: Firenze University Press; 2019. p. 195–7. ISSN: 978-88-6453-961-4.
24. Pedersen M, Agersted A, Akram B, Mahmood S, Jønsson A, Mahmood S. Optical coherence tomography in the laryngeal arytenoid mucosa for documentation of pharmacological treatments and genetic aspects: a protocol. Adv Cell Mol Otolaryngol. 2016;4(1):32246. https://doi.org/10.3402/acmo.v4.32246.
25. Wong BJ, Jackson RP, Guo S, Ridgway JM, Mahmood U, Su J, et al. In vivo optical coherence tomography of the human larynx: normative and benign pathology in 82 patients. Laryngoscope. 2005;115(11):1904–11. https://doi.org/10.1097/01.MLG.0000181465.17744.BE. Erratum in: Laryngoscope 2006;116(3):507.
26. Klein AM, Pierce MC, Zeitels SM, Anderson RR, Kobler JB, Shishkov M, de Boer JF. Imaging the human vocal folds in vivo with optical coherence tomography: a preliminary experience. Ann Otol Rhinol Laryngol. 2006;115(4):277–84. https://doi.org/10.1177/000348940611500405.

27. Burns JA, Kim KH, Anderson RR. Laryngeal imaging with polarization-sensitive optical coherence tomography. Proc SPIE. 2011;7883:78832N. https://doi.org/10.1117/12.875443.
28. Mongeau L. The 13th international conference on advances in quantitative laryngology, voice and speech research (June 2–4, 2019, Montreal, Quebec, Canada). Appl Sci. 2019;9(13):2665. https://doi.org/10.3390/app9132665.
29. Yu L, Liu G, Rubinstein M, Saidi A, Wong BJ, Chen Z. Office-based dynamic imaging of vocal cords in awake patients with swept-source optical coherence tomography. J Biomed Opt. 2009;14(6):064020. https://doi.org/10.1117/1.3268442.
30. Garcia JA, Benboujja F, Beaudette K, Guo R, Boudoux C, Hartnick CJ. Using attenuation coefficients from optical coherence tomography as markers of vocal fold maturation. Laryngoscope. 2016;126(6):E218–23. https://doi.org/10.1002/lary.25765.
31. Garcia JA. Attenuation coefficients, pixel intensity, and texture analysis as quantitative parameters for analyzing optical coherence tomography images of vocal fold tissue [dissertation on the Internet]. Boston: Harvard Medical School; 2016. Available from: http://nrs.harvard.edu/urn-3:HUL.InstRepos:27007738.
32. Benboujja F, Greenberg M, Nourmahnad A, Rath N, Hartnick C. Evaluation of the human vocal fold lamina propria development using optical coherence tomography. Laryngoscope. 2021;131(9):E2558–65. https://doi.org/10.1002/lary.29516.
33. Benboujja F, Hartnick C. Publisher correction: Quantitative evaluation of the human vocal fold extracellular matrix using multiphoton microscopy and optical coherence tomography. Sci Rep. 2021;11(1):4752. https://doi.org/10.1038/s41598-021-84391-7. Erratum for: Sci Rep 2021;11(1):2440. doi: 10.1038/s41598-021-82157-9.
34. Bang O, Jain D, Petersen CR, Israelsen NM, Markos C. Optical coherence tomography system. US Patent App. 17/283,224. 2020.
35. Vestri G, Macaluso C, Versaci F. Anterior segment OCT: fundamentals and technological basis. In: Essentials in ophthalmology/essentials ophthalmology. Cham: Springer; 2020. p. 5–19. https://doi.org/10.1007/978-3-030-53374-8_2.
36. Israelsen N, Larsen CF, Pedersen M. Kvantitativ undersøgelse af stemmebånd med højhastighedsvideo og optisk kohærens-tomografi. Ugeskr Læger. 2022;184:V02210146. Also published in European Voice Teachers Association (EVTA) Echo #2 – May 2023 in English.
37. Coughlan CA, Chou LD, Jing JC, Chen JJ, Rangarajan S, Chang TH, et al. In vivo cross-sectional imaging of the phonating larynx using long-range Doppler optical coherence tomography. Sci Rep. 2016;6:22792. https://doi.org/10.1038/srep22792.
38. Meller A, Shakhova M, Rilkin Y, Novozhilov A, Kirillin M, Shakhov A. Optical coherence tomography in diagnosing inflammatory diseases of ENT. Photonics Lasers Med. 2014;3(4):323–30. https://doi.org/10.1515/plm-2014-0025.
39. Sharma GK, Chen LY, Chou L, Badger C, Hong E, Rangarajan S, et al. Surface kinematic and depth-resolved analysis of human vocal folds in vivo during phonation using optical coherence tomography. J Biomed Opt. 2021;26(8):086005. https://doi.org/10.1117/1.JBO.26.8.086005.
40. Wittig L, Betz C, Eggert D. Optical coherence tomography for tissue classification of the larynx in an outpatient setting-a translational challenge on the verge of a resolution? Transl Biophotonics. 2020;3(1):e202000013. https://doi.org/10.1002/tbio.202000013.
41. Wei W, Choi WJ, Men S, Song S, Wang RK. Wide-field and long-ranging-depth optical coherence tomography microangiography of human oral mucosa. Proc SPIE. 2018;10473:104730H. https://doi.org/10.1117/12.2290685.
42. Pham TT, Chen L, Heidari AE, Chen JJ, Zhukhovitskaya A, Li Y, et al. Computational analysis of six optical coherence tomography systems for vocal fold imaging: a comparison study. Lasers Surg Med. 2019;51(5):412–22. https://doi.org/10.1002/lsm.23060.
43. Gessert N, Schlüter M, Latus S, Volgger V, Betz C, Schlaefer A. Towards automatic lesion classification in the upper aerodigestive tract using OCT and deep transfer learning methods. arXiv:1902.03618. 2019. https://doi.org/10.48550/arXiv.1902.03618.
44. Mahmood U, Ridgway J, Jackson R, Guo S, Su J, Armstrong W, et al. In vivo optical coherence tomography of the nasal mucosa. Am J Rhinol. 2006;20(2):155–9. https://doi.org/10.1177/194589240602000206.

45. Pedersen M, Larsen CF, Madsen B, Eeg M. Localization and quantification of glottal gaps on deep learning segmentation of vocal folds. Sci Rep. 2023;13(1):878. https://doi.org/10.1038/s41598-023-27980-y.
46. Roth DF, Abbott KV, Carroll TL, Ferguson BJ. Evidence for primary laryngeal inhalant allergy: a randomized, double-blinded crossover study. Int Forum Allergy Rhinol. 2013;3(1):10–8. https://doi.org/10.1002/alr.21051.

Open Access This chapter is licensed under the terms of the Creative Commons Attribution-NonCommercial-NoDerivatives 4.0 International License (http://creativecommons.org/licenses/by-nc-nd/4.0/), which permits any noncommercial use, sharing, distribution and reproduction in any medium or format, as long as you give appropriate credit to the original author(s) and the source, provide a link to the Creative Commons license and indicate if you modified the licensed material. You do not have permission under this license to share adapted material derived from this chapter or parts of it.

The images or other third party material in this chapter are included in the chapter's Creative Commons license, unless indicated otherwise in a credit line to the material. If material is not included in the chapter's Creative Commons license and your intended use is not permitted by statutory regulation or exceeds the permitted use, you will need to obtain permission directly from the copyright holder.

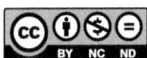

Overview and Conclusion

Mette Pedersen, Neveen Hassan Nashaat, Ramón Hernández-Villoria, Valentina Camesasca, and Sneha Das

The book is divided into two parts: the first focuses on methods, while the second explores clinical applications.

Biomarkers are objective and quantifiable characteristics of biological processes that can predict disease outcomes. In the introduction chapter of the Committee on Biomarkers in Phoniatrics, the potential applications of voice-related biomarkers are discussed. These biomarkers must consider the glottis's closure three key functions: breathing, phonation, and airway protection during swallowing.

Voice-related biomarkers are measurable features of the voice that are linked to clinical outcomes, enabling health monitoring, diagnosis, and disease severity assessment. The rapid advancement of digital technologies, particularly during the global pandemic, has expanded the use of voice-related biomarkers due to their noninvasive, accessible, and cost-effective collection through digital devices.

M. Pedersen (✉)
The Medical Center, Copenhagen, Denmark
e-mail: M.f.pedersen@dadlnet.dk

N. Hassan Nashaat
Research on Children with Special Needs Department, Medical Research and Clinical Studies Institute, National Research Centre, Cairo, Egypt

R. Hernández-Villoria
Centro Clínico de Audición y Lenguaje Cealca, Caracas, Venezuela

Hospital de Clínicas Caracas, Caracas, Venezuela

V. Camesasca
Grande Ospedale Metropolitano Niguarda, Centro Clinico NEMO (NeuroMuscolar Omnicenter), Milano, Italy

S. Das
Technical University of Denmark, Kongens Lyngby, Denmark

Pioneer Centre for Artificial Intelligence, Copenhagen, Denmark

The Union of European Phoniatricians' Biomarker Committee aims to advance knowledge of digital technologies, identify characteristic voice features across various disorders, and define accessible parameters with the potential to serve as biomarkers of glottal closure. Self-assessment using the Voice Handicap Index, clinical evaluation with GRBAS tests, analysis of acoustic parameters—including fundamental frequency (F0), jitter, shimmer, and harmonics-to-noise ratio (HNR)—and maximal phonation time (MPT) are key components of voice diagnostics. However, a significant limitation remains: no voice-related digital biomarkers have been approved by the FDA to date.

Two literature searches were conducted by The Royal Society of Medicine Library (UK) covering the period from 2013 to 2023. The results highlighted Parkinson's disease as the leading disorder for which usable voice-related biomarkers were identified as a viable option.

Accordingly, an overview of voice-related parameters in Parkinson's disease was presented, discussing aspects of biomarkers through a review of the literature, along with measurement methods utilized both with and without machine learning.

Although the literature review primarily centers on Parkinson's disease, the findings likely have broader implications, suggesting that the analysis could be applicable to a variety of voice-related conditions.

14.1 Analysis for Neurologic Diseases

Artificial intelligence (AI) has been successfully utilized for voice analysis to identify and classify patients with disorders such as Parkinson's disease, Alzheimer's disease, and multiple sclerosis. AI is emerging as a promising tool for the early detection, staging, and monitoring of the progression of these conditions. The presented models for the success of AI-enhanced voice analysis lie in the computerized programs used for analysis and the carefully selected AI tools designed for learning, which help clinicians optimize patient management strategies.

AI-enhanced voice analysis, particularly through Deep Learning (DL) models, will in the future offer the advantages of being cost-effective, noninvasive, and adaptable to cross-language differences. Future advancements in extracting voice parameters from speech using AI will largely depend on a deeper understanding of the relationship between connected speech and specific voice parameters.

However, at present, the sensitivity and specificity of these methods remain suboptimal, highlighting the need for further research and development to improve their accuracy and reliability.

Parkinson's disease is used as a primary example, as previous voice analyses, including those utilizing AI models, have primarily focused on the voice-related aspects of this disorder. How can all factors be contextualized within the framework of the disorder, providing a comprehensive understanding of their relevance? Acoustic, perceptual, aerodynamic, and self-assessment factors of the voice, along with associated risk factors and confounding factors that need to be excluded to build a model.

14.2 Automatic Classification of Diseases from Speech and Voice

Glottal inverse filtering is a technique used to estimate the glottal volume velocity waveform, which is the source of voiced speech, from the speech pressure signal recorded by a microphone. Glottal parameters, when combined with machine learning and deep learning classifiers, can automatically detect diseases and classify their severity based on speech signals. Despite its clinical significance and practical usability, this method remains underutilized for reasons that are not well understood.

Glottal inverse filtering holds particular interest because it defines glottal closure, making airflow analysis another key aspect. In pathology, numerous parameters derived from this technique are valuable, particularly in the lower register of voice, as discussed in detail in the fifth chapter of this book.

A key aspect of the fundamental building blocks of AI systems—data, model types, and evaluation—is the critical factor necessary for the successful deployment of voice-AI in clinical settings, particularly reproducibility and trust. The various AI models have to be thoroughly assessed to ensure their applicability and reliability.

An important quality consideration is the diversity and representation of the subjects within the dataset. For example, before deploying automatic GBRBAS assessment tools, it is essential to consider factors such as age, gender, and other characteristics of the expected user population. This also extends our understanding of the hierarchical associations between the data samples.

Furthermore, various software models applying machine learning to specific voice-related biomarkers have been explored, highlighting their potential for advancing voice diagnostics and clinical applications.

14.3 Voice-Related Biomarkers

Biomarkers must hold both prognostic/predictive and monetary values. While this may seem straightforward, the interpretation and application of voice-related biomarkers in medical contexts are complex, encompassing phonation, ventilation, airway protection, and their integration with artificial intelligence (AI). By definition, a biomarker must fulfill at least three fundamental criteria: specificity, effectiveness, and efficiency. In the field of phoniatrics, a distinction is made between sound production, which occurs at the level of the vocal folds, and the audible outcome—speech—which is influenced by resonator and articulatory factors as the sound passes through the vocal tract. Furthermore, phoniatrics differentiates between speech and language, with the latter involving higher-level cognitive processes such as word finding, rhythm, and prosody.

Glottal Inverse Filtering (GIF) has numerous applications across various fields, including artificial voice production, such as converting text to voice. For the study of the aerodynamics of the glottal function, GIF is possible through very simple and friendly software. A second-level application of GIF incorporates the theory of operation of the phonatory source as a three-mass system.

An in-depth review of the three apps' key tools used for these analyses—Aalto Aparat, Sopran, and the Online Lab Voice Clinical System. It discusses their features, strengths, and limitations, offering insights into their roles in evaluating specific voice biomarkers and their broader clinical applications.

Aspects of software tools were discussed. The quality of the results was completely dependent on the dataset. Once the dataset, features, metrics, and reproducibility are well defined, the quality of testing, evaluation, and validation is also important. Thereafter, the impact of system performance on patient outcomes was assessed, before large-scale deployment of voice-biomarker AI models/software in hospitals and clinics, randomized controlled trials should be considered.

14.4 Pathology of Voice-Related Biomarkers in Laryngology and in Neurodegenerative Diseases

Laryngeal disorders and voice-related biomarkers were discussed. Voice-related biomarkers are variables that serve as monitors of laryngeal pathologies. They rely on clinicians, patients, and devices. Changes in voice-related biomarkers will help clinicians in their voice health plans for laryngeal disorders.

On the other hand, neurodegenerative disorders and voice-related biomarkers were explored. Several studies show promising results regarding possible voice-related digital biomarkers with traditional acoustic measures. Neurotechnologies, such as automatic voice analyzers and speech recognition systems, are based on artificial intelligence. These methods may be useful to identify subtle preclinical voice impairments in neurodegenerative disorders.

14.5 Genetics and the Application of Voice-Related Biomarkers

In genetics, a new perspective is emerging that voice diagnostics and treatment may assist patients in improving their communication with their surroundings. This raises the question of whether voice-related biomarkers are used. A literature search revealed that voice-related biomarkers are being utilized, and their use has increased in recent studies. However, most authors noted that their findings were among the first of their kind in the literature and that, in many cases, only a single voice-related biomarker was employed.

Looking forward, the UEP committee recommends incorporating all four suggested biomarkers into future studies, potentially as part of a voice foundation model.

The limitations of this chapter include the inability to categorize genetic disorders into distinct groups, as studies involving voice-related biomarkers have thus far appeared sporadically across various genetic disorder groups.

14.6 Optical Coherence Tomography and Voice-Related Biomarkers

In recent years, there has been a growing emphasis on the noninvasive nature of biomarkers, which is why techniques such as endoscopy, including optical coherence tomography (OCT), have not been extensively evaluated until now. Endoscopic methods utilizing OCT provide a detailed evaluation of tissue structures, forming a foundation for further studies at the genetic level.

A key advantage of this method is its ability to measure vocal fold function at the cellular level. Looking ahead, the integration of machine learning into endoscopy techniques is expected to make OCT more accessible and efficient, reducing the challenges typically associated with invasive methods. As such, the potential of OCT as a voice-related biomarker cannot be disregarded.

While limitations such as the complexity of endoscopic procedures remain significant, future efforts will likely focus on overcoming these challenges to fully realize the potential of OCT and similar technologies in voice diagnostics and research.

14.7 Voice-Related Biomarkers and AI: A Very Near Future?

In the context of the growing impact of the development of artificial intelligence methods and their orientation towards more effective ways of detecting health problems at stages in which they barely produce symptoms for those with the problem, the study of voice-related biomarkers will acquire great relevance.

This relevance will be due to the ease of registration, usability, wide dissemination of both software and hardware worldwide, and the consequent very low costs that this has for both developers and end users.

The strategies for focusing on the results obtained through devices aimed at the early detection of, for example, Parkinson's disease, will guide towards concrete actions that will allow the contact of the detected people with the health systems in an early and therefore very advantageous way.

Understanding the human voice as a multidimensional phenomenon, whose actual quality depends on the interrelation between systems and many factors, will be crucial to achieving development in the precision of designed AI-based tools.

It is important to rethink the taxonomy of biomarkers as the use of voice-related biomarkers expands. It is important to highlight that voice-related biomarkers whose consistency and correspondence with pathologies of the larynx, respiratory tract, or cardiovascular system have been demonstrated and categorized by a multitude of studies, should be subjected to correlation analysis.

The integration of biomarkers related to the voice in the different practical tools that are proposed for detection and diagnosis purposes within phoniatrics or outside it will, in any case, have to be subject to a theoretical construct that explains the outputs obtained: a health-disease model will always be needed, whether the focus is a pathology of the vocal cords, a neurodegenerative disorder, a mental disease, or heart failure.

The stages of evolution of the glottal inverse filter or traditional acoustic voice analysis methods are leading on the path to an increasingly successful integration between them, precisely because they explore different extractable aspects of the vocal sound, whether these are aerodynamic or directly related to the physics of the complex soundwave of the phonatory source.

When these analytical techniques are framed in a model of the functioning of a biological system that they aim to account for, the resulting tool acquires much more power than simply obtaining isolated data allows us to deduce.

In the near future, areas such as endocrinology and immunology could, in a much cheaper way than that provided by blood-based laboratory means or imaging means, obtain rapid and early answers regarding subtle changes in functioning.

For doctors specializing in phoniatrics or for scientists interested in the phoniatric applications of biomarkers related to the voice, the discovery and progressive development of these will expand their fields of action and research. Will they be replaced at some point by machines capable of replacing their role? It is possible, but in the meantime, it is inevitable to join its evolution by guiding the paths to be followed.

Open Access This chapter is licensed under the terms of the Creative Commons Attribution-NonCommercial-NoDerivatives 4.0 International License (http://creativecommons.org/licenses/by-nc-nd/4.0/), which permits any noncommercial use, sharing, distribution and reproduction in any medium or format, as long as you give appropriate credit to the original author(s) and the source, provide a link to the Creative Commons license and indicate if you modified the licensed material. You do not have permission under this license to share adapted material derived from this chapter or parts of it.

The images or other third party material in this chapter are included in the chapter's Creative Commons license, unless indicated otherwise in a credit line to the material. If material is not included in the chapter's Creative Commons license and your intended use is not permitted by statutory regulation or exceeds the permitted use, you will need to obtain permission directly from the copyright holder.

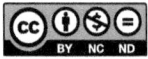

GPSR Compliance

The European Union's (EU) General Product Safety Regulation (GPSR) is a set of rules that requires consumer products to be safe and our obligations to ensure this.

If you have any concerns about our products, you can contact us on ProductSafety@springernature.com

In case Publisher is established outside the EU, the EU authorized representative is:

Springer Nature Customer Service Center GmbH
Europaplatz 3
69115 Heidelberg, Germany

Batch number: 09458182

Printed by Printforce, the Netherlands